Testimonials from the
GLUCOSE GODDESS
Instagram Community

While these testimonials are based on individual success stories, results may vary.

"A few days of applying Jessie's tips and my cravings disappeared. That changed everything." —*Laura, 63*

"I'm eating pasta and losing weight. How much more awesome does it get?" —*Jasmin, 20*

"After two years of not ovulating, I'm regularly ovulating again. I lost 35 pounds. My acne cleared up. And mentally I am feeling so much better. The information Jessie shares changed my life. No going back!" —*Heather, 31*

"Jessie has shown me that I could change how menopause went for me. My friends told me I would never be able to lose the weight I had gained. Thanks to Jessie I proved them wrong! With her glucose hacks, I lost 9 pounds, I sleep like I used to, I feel amazing, and I no longer want to nap in the middle of the afternoon. I feel even better than before menopause." —*Bernadette, 55*

"I was diagnosed with type 2 diabetes after my third pregnancy 16 years ago. For years it's been getting worse and it's been difficult to manage. After starting to implement Jessie's hacks, in four months, I went from 200 mg/dL fasting glucose level to 110 mg/dL: from severely diabetic to diabetic no longer. I've been able to reverse the condition on my own!" —*Fatemeh, 51*

"Life-changing information . . . I lost 36 pounds in two months! My recurrent migraine problem improved significantly, and my energy is through the roof. I feel better than ever."   —*Annalaura, 49*

"In four months of following Jessie's glucose teachings, I've effortlessly lost 13 pounds, my massive hormonal acne is gone, and for the first time in my adult life I have normal thyroid levels (I went from 8.7 mIU/L TSH to 4.4 mIU/L). I have never felt better."   —*Tamara, 31*

"I'm a 64-year-old breast cancer survivor with heart, glucose, and thyroid conditions. I take hormone suppressors and yet I have managed to lose 18 pounds in three months with the ridiculously easy changes Jessie explains so well. I'm the slimmest I've been since I gave birth and my blood tests are, in the words of my doctor, 'those of a 15-year-old.' It's hard to believe, even for me! Thank you, Jessie, for changing my life."
          —*Dovra, 64*

"I'm a type 1 diabetic. I used to spike up to 300 mg/dL after breakfast. With the information Jessie shares I've learned to keep my glucose steady and my HbA1c has dropped from 7.4 percent to 5.1 percent in three months . . . I don't snap at my family and friends anymore. I can finally be the person I want to be."   —*Lucy, 24*

"I have no words to describe how much Jessie's hacks changed my life. Two years ago I stopped taking the pill with the aim of starting a family. I thought it would be easy. But my period never came. After a year, I went to the doctor. I was diagnosed with insulin resistance and PCOS. It was really hard. Thankfully I found Jessie's work and I had hope again . . . I started implementing her tips. My period came back after two months! All my PCOS symptoms vanished (hair growth, anxiety, constant eating) and now . . . I have just found out I'm pregnant! I'm so happy I cannot describe it!"   —*Filipa, 29*

"I went from 19 percent body fat percentage to 8 percent. So happy! And all this while eating all the foods I love."   —*Semir, 24*

"I was diagnosed with gestational diabetes at 29 weeks pregnant. So far, after one month of Jessie's tips, huge changes: I feel better than I ever did during the pregnancy, I'm not swollen, my blood sugar levels are steady and managed, my doctor is happy, and, most importantly, I'm not scared anymore. Can't recommend Jessie's work enough for all moms-to-be."
—*Paulina, 39*

"I've been severely bulimic for nearly 30 years and nothing had ever helped until I started following Jessie and taking care of my glucose levels with her hacks. I haven't binged or purged for two months now, which is unbelievable. I honestly thought it was something that was just a part of me and I would never get over."
—*Sue, 48*

"I've dealt with hypoglycemia (low blood sugar) for a number of years. I was unaware that I could significantly improve it by just changing a few things about how I ate, like the order in which to eat my food. Thanks to Jessie and her evidence-based observations, I've learned how to eat a cookie or chocolate with far fewer negative impacts. Now that my blood sugar is more stable, I'm able to better address my anxiety symptoms and focus on dealing with its root causes."
—*Ilana, 37*

"In one month I feel like I've been reborn. I've had myalgic enceph-alomyelitis and chronic fatigue most of my life. I have also struggled with long Covid symptoms. After discovering Glucose Goddess, I feel so much better—I'm healthier, happier, and my energy is back! A huge thank-you."
—*Christie, 37*

"Over the last two years my hair was falling out like crazy. I was con-fused and devastated. And then a miracle happened: I followed the Glu-cose Goddess principles for 40 days and now it's growing back fuller and thicker! I am so happy! Not just that, but I've reversed my predia-betes too (I used to have 110 mg/dL fasting glucose levels, now they are 96). My energy is so much more stable during the day, and my hunger and thirst levels too. I no longer need that second cup of coffee in the afternoon or that 'emergency' snack. My mental clarity has improved and my adult acne went away. It's amazing how quickly the changes happened. I recommend Jessie to everyone I know."   —*Aya, 27*

"I have type 1 diabetes. For decades no one could help me with it. Since discovering Glucose Goddess, my cravings disappeared, I was finally able to follow a healthier diet, and my glucose went from 530 mg/dL to 156 in the first days and my insulin dose divided by 10. Oh, and I lost 6 pounds! My doctor and nutritionist were so surprised and now they recommend Glucose Goddess to their patients."   —*Mariel, 43*

GLUCOSE REVOLUTION

Stop Cravings, Get Your Energy Back, Feel Amazing, and Still Eat What You Love

The Life-Changing Power of Balancing Your Blood Sugar

~~~~~

JESSIE INCHAUSPÉ

Simon & Schuster

New York   London   Toronto   Sydney   New Delhi

Simon & Schuster
1230 Avenue of the Americas
New York, NY 10020

First Simon & Schuster hardcover edition April 2022

SIMON & SCHUSTER and colophon are registered
trademarks of Simon & Schuster, Inc.

For information about special discounts for bulk
purchases, please contact Simon & Schuster Special Sales at
1-866-506-1949 or business@simonandschuster.com.

The Simon & Schuster Speakers Bureau can bring authors to your
live event. For more information or to book an event, contact
the Simon & Schuster Speakers Bureau at 1-866-248-3049
or visit our website at www.simonspeakers.com.

Interior design by Lewelin Polanco

Manufactured in the United States of America

9 10 8

Library of Congress Control Number: 202195045

ISBN 978-1-9821-7941-0
ISBN 978-1-9821-7943-4 (ebook)

Contents

PART 3: HOW CAN I FLATTEN MY GLUCOSE CURVES?

To my family

Dear Reader

What was the last thing you ate?

Go on, think about it for a second.

Did you like it? What did it look like? What did it smell like? What did it taste like? Where were you when you ate it? Who were you with? And why did you pick it?

Food is not only delicious, it is vital to us. Yet sometimes, without our knowing, food can also cause unintended consequences. So now for the harder questions: Do you know how many grams of fat were added to your belly after eating that thing? Do you know if it will cause you to wake up with a pimple tomorrow? Do you know how much plaque it built up in your arteries or how many wrinkles it deepened on your face? Do you know if it's the reason you'll be hungry again in two hours, sleep poorly tonight, or feel sluggish tomorrow?

In short—do you know what the last thing you ate did to your body and mind?

Many of us don't. I certainly didn't before I started learning about a molecule called glucose.

For most of us, our body is a black box: we know its function but not exactly how it works. We often decide what to have for lunch based on what we read or hear, rather than based on what our bodies truly need.

"The animal tends to eat with his stomach, and the man with his brain," wrote the philosopher Alan Watts. If only our bodies could speak to us, it would be a different story. We'd know exactly why we were hungry again in two hours, why we slept poorly last night, and why we felt sluggish the next day. We would make better decisions about what we ate. Our health would improve. Our lives would improve.

Well, I've got a scoop for you.

As it turns out, our bodies speak to us all the time.

We just don't know how to listen.

Everything we put in our mouth creates a reaction. What we eat affects the 30 trillion cells and 30 trillion bacteria within us. Take your pick: cravings, pimples, migraines, brain fog, mood swings, weight gain, sleepiness, infertility, polycystic ovarian syndrome (PCOS), type 2 diabetes, fatty liver disease, heart disease . . . are all messages from our bodies that there are problems within.

This is where I blame our environment. Our nutritional choices are influenced by billion-dollar marketing campaigns aimed at making money for the food industry—campaigns for soda, fast food, and candy. These are usually justified under the guise of "what matters is how much you eat—processed foods and sugar aren't inherently bad." But science is demonstrating the opposite: processed foods and sugar *are* inherently bad for us, even if we don't eat them in caloric excess.

Even so, it's because of this misleading marketing that we believe statements such as:

"Weight loss is just about calories in and calories out."

"You should never skip breakfast."

"Rice cakes and fruit juice are good for you."

"Fatty foods are bad for you."

"You need to eat sugar to have energy."

"Type 2 diabetes is a genetic disease that you can't do anything about."

"If you aren't losing weight, it's because you don't have enough willpower."

"Feeling sleepy at 3 p.m. is normal—drink some coffee."

Our misled food choices influence our physical and mental well-being—and stop us from waking up every morning feeling amazing. It may not seem like much that we don't feel amazing every morning, but if you could . . . wouldn't you? I'm here to tell you there's a way you can.

Scientists have been studying how food affects us for a long time, and we now know more than we ever have on this topic. Exciting discoveries have happened in the past five years in labs around the world: they've revealed our body's reaction to food *in real time*—and have proven that although *what* we eat matters, *how* we eat it—in which order, combination, and grouping—matters, too.

What the science shows is that in the black box that is our body, there is one metric that affects all systems. If we understand this one metric and make choices to optimize it, we can greatly improve our physical and mental well-being. This metric is the amount of blood sugar, or *glucose*, in our blood.

Glucose is our body's main source of energy. We get most of it from the food we eat, and it's then carried in our bloodstream to our cells. Its concentration can fluctuate greatly throughout the day, and sharp increases in concentration—I call them *glucose spikes*—affect everything from our mood, our sleep, our weight, and our skin to the health of our immune system, our risk for heart disease, and our chance of conception.

You will rarely hear glucose discussed unless you have diabetes, but glucose actually affects each and every one of us. In the last few years, the tools to monitor this molecule have become more readily available. That, in combination with the advancements in science I mentioned above, means that we have access to more data than ever before—and we can use those data to gain insight into our bodies.

This book is organized into three parts: (1) what glucose is and what we mean when we talk about glucose spikes, (2) why glucose spikes are harmful, and (3) what we can do to avoid spikes while still eating the food we love.

In part 1, I explain what glucose is, where it comes from, and why it's so important. The science is out there, but the news isn't spreading nearly fast enough. Regulating glucose is important for everyone, diabetes or no diabetes: 88 percent of Americans are likely to have dysregulated glucose levels (even if they are not overweight according to medical guidelines), and most don't know it. When our glucose levels are dysregulated, we experience glucose spikes. During a spike, glucose floods into our body quickly, increasing its concentration in our bloodstream by more than 30 milligrams per deciliter (mg/dL) in the span of about an hour (or less), then decreasing just as quickly. The spikes lead to harmful consequences.

In part 2, I describe how glucose spikes affect us in the short term—hunger, cravings, fatigue, worse menopause symptoms, migraine, poor sleep, difficulty managing type 1 diabetes and gestational diabetes, weakened immune system, worsened cognitive function— and in the long term. Dysregulated glucose levels contribute to aging and to the development of chronic diseases such as acne, eczema, psoriasis, arthritis, cataracts, Alzheimer's disease, cancer, depression, gut problems, heart disease, infertility, PCOS, insulin resistance, type 2 diabetes, and fatty liver disease.

If you were to plot your glucose level every minute of every day on a graph, the line between the points would have peaks and valleys. That graph would show your *glucose curve*. When we make lifestyle changes to avoid spikes, we flatten our glucose curves. The flatter our glucose curves, the better. With flatter glucose curves, we reduce the amount of insulin—a hormone released in response to glucose—in our body, and this is beneficial, as too much insulin is one of the main drivers of insulin resistance, type 2 diabetes, and PCOS. With flatter glucose curves, we also naturally flatten our fructose curves—fructose is found alongside glucose in sugary foods—which is also beneficial, as too much fructose increases the likelihood of obesity, heart disease, and nonalcoholic fatty liver disease.

In part 3, I'll show you how you can flatten your glucose curves with 10 simple food hacks that you can easily incorporate into your life. I studied mathematics in college, then biochemistry in grad school, and this training has allowed me to analyze and distill a vast amount of nutritional science. In addition, I have run many experiments on myself wearing a device called a continuous glucose monitor, which shows me my glucose levels in real time. These 10 hacks I will share are simple and surprising. None asks you to never eat dessert again, count calories, or exercise for hours and hours a day. Instead, they ask you to use what you've learned about your physiology in parts I and II—really listening to your body—to make better decisions about *how* you eat. (And that often means putting *more* food on our plate than usual.) In this final section, I will arm you with all the information you'll need to avoid glucose spikes without wearing a monitor yourself.

Throughout this book, I draw on cutting-edge science to explain why these hacks work and tell real-life stories that show them in action. You will see data taken from my own experiments and experiments from the Glucose Goddess community, an online community I have built and grown that has (at printing time) over 200,000 members. And you'll read testimonials from members who have shed weight, curbed their cravings, improved their energy, cleared their skin, rid themselves of PCOS symptoms, reversed type 2 diabetes, done away with guilt, and gained immense self-confidence based on the insights here.

By the end of this book, you'll be able to listen to the messages coming from your body—and understand what to do next. You'll make empowered food decisions, no longer prey to marketing messages. Your health will improve, and so will your life.

I know this for a fact because it happened to me.

How I Got Here

You know the saying "Don't take your health for granted"? Well, I did, until an accident at 19 changed my life.

I was in Hawaii on vacation with friends. One afternoon we went for a hike in the jungle, and we decided that jumping off a waterfall would be a great idea (spoiler alert: it was not).

It was the first time I had ever tried anything like it. My friends had told me what to do: "Keep your legs really straight so that your feet go into the water first."

"Got it!" I said, and off I went.

Totally terrified, I forgot that advice as soon as I leapt off the edge of the cliff. I did *not* land feet first—I landed butt first. The pressure from the water created a shock wave up my spine, and, like dominos falling, each of my vertebrae compressed.

Shack-shack-shack-shack-shack-shack-shack, they went—all the way up to my second thoracic vertebra, which exploded into fourteen pieces under the pressure.

My life exploded into pieces, too. After that, I divided it in two: *before* the accident and *after* the accident.

I spent the next two weeks immobilized in a hospital bed, waiting to undergo spinal surgery. As I lay awake, I kept mentally picturing what was going to happen, unable to fully believe it: the surgeon was going to open my torso from the side, at my waist, then from the back, at the level of the broken vertebra. He was going to take out the bone fragments as well as the two surrounding disks, then fuse three vertebrae together and drill six three-inch metal rods into my spine. With an *electric drill*.

The risks associated with the procedure terrified me: lung perforation, paralysis, and death. It wasn't as though I had a choice, though. The vertebral pieces were pressing against the membrane of my spinal cord. Any shock (even tripping on a stair) could lead them to rupture the membrane, paralyzing me from the waist down. I was scared. I imagined myself on the operating table, bleeding out, and the doctors giving up. I imagined my life ending like that, all because I had gotten scared in midair doing something that was supposed to be fun.

The day of the surgery approached slowly but surely, though when it finally arrived, I wished it hadn't. As the anesthesiologist

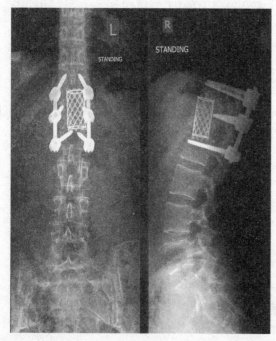

The finished result. (No, I don't set off the alarm at airport security, and yes, this stays in forever.)

began putting me under for the eight-hour procedure, I wondered if she would be the last person I ever saw. I prayed. I wanted to live. If I could wake up on the other side of this, I knew I would be filled with gratitude for the rest of my life.

~~~~~

I woke up. It was the middle of the night, and I was alone in a recovery room. At first, I felt immense relief: I was alive. Then I felt pain. Correction: I felt a *lot* of pain. The new hardware was like an iron fist squeezing my spine. I tried to sit up to call a nurse. After a few tries he showed up, moody and dismissive. It was a dismal way to be greeted back into the world. I cried. I just wanted my mom.

It's true, I was filled with gratitude: deep, profound gratitude to be alive. But I was also in agony. My entire back was throbbing, I couldn't move an inch without feeling that my stitches were going to rip open, and the nerves in my legs were on fire for days. I was allowed a shot of painkillers every three hours. Like clockwork, a nurse would come into my room, pinch the fat on my thigh, and administer the needle—alternating legs each time. I couldn't sleep because everything hurt so much, nor eat because the opioids made me nauseous. I lost 25 pounds in two weeks. I felt at once lucky and stupid, sorry for what had happened, guilty for putting my loved ones through this, and at a loss for what to do.

My body healed in a matter of months, but then my mind and soul were the ones that needed rehab. I felt disconnected from reality. When I looked at my hands, they didn't seem like mine. When I looked in the mirror, I was terrified. Something was wrong. But I didn't know what.

Unfortunately, no one else did, either. From the outside I seemed well again. So I kept my suffering to myself. When someone asked me how I was, I answered, "I'm great, thanks." If I was being honest, though, I would have responded, "I feel like a stranger in my own body, I can't look in the mirror without losing my mind, and I'm scared to death that I'm never going to be okay again." That was later diagnosed as depersonalization-derealization disorder, a mental disorder where people can't connect to themselves or the reality around them.

I was living in London at the time, and I remember sitting in the Tube, looking at the commuters opposite me, wondering how many of them were also going through something difficult and hiding it, just like I was. I dreamed that someone on the train would recognize my suffering and tell me that they understood—that they had felt as I had and come back to themselves. But of course, in vain. The people sitting three feet away had no idea what was going on inside me. *I* barely knew what was going on inside me. And I had no idea what was going on inside them and whether or not they were suffering, too.

It became abundantly clear to me that it's hard to know what is going on inside our bodies. Even when we can give voice to our emotions—gratitude, pain, relief, sadness, and more—we must then find out why. Where do we start when we don't feel okay?

I remember telling my best friend, "Nothing matters—not school, not work, not money—nothing matters more than being healthy, physically and mentally." It was the deepest conviction I had ever felt.

~~~~~

And that was how, four years later, I ended up on the train headed thirty-nine miles south of San Francisco, to an office in Mountain View. Having decided to figure out how to communicate with my body, I felt that I needed to work at the forefront of health technology. In 2015, that forefront was genetics.

I had landed an internship at the startup 23andMe (so named because we all have twenty-three pairs of chromosomes that carry our genetic code). And I wanted to be there more than I had ever wanted to be anywhere.

My thinking went like this: My DNA created my body, so if I can understand my DNA, I can understand my body.

I worked as a product manager. I had two degrees under my belt and a passion for making complicated subjects simple. I was putting those to good use: I was in charge of explaining genetic research to our customers and encouraging them to participate by answering surveys. We collected data as it had never been done before: digitally, online, on millions of people at once. Each customer was a citizen scientist, contributing to advancing our collective understanding of DNA. The goal was to innovate in the field of personalized medicine and deliver health recommendations unique to each individual.

It was the best place, with the best people, the best data, and the best mission. The atmosphere at the office was electric.

I grew close to the other scientists on the research team, then read through all the papers they had published and started asking questions. But to my disappointment, little by little, it became clear to me that DNA wasn't as predictive as I had thought. For instance, your genes can increase your likelihood of developing type 2 diabetes, but they can't tell you for sure whether you'll get it. Looking at your DNA can only give you a sense of what *might* happen. For most chronic conditions, from migraines to heart disease, the cause ends up being much more attributable to "lifestyle factors" than to genetics. In short, your genes don't determine how you feel when you wake up in the morning.

In 2018, 23andMe launched a new initiative. It was led by the Health Research & Development team, which was in charge of coming up with cutting-edge ideas. They were discussing . . . *continuous glucose monitors*.

Continuous glucose monitors (CGMs) are small devices worn on the back of your arm that track glucose levels. They were created to replace the finger pricks that people with diabetes have been using for decades and that give glucose measurements only a few times a day. With a CGM, glucose levels are measured every few minutes.

Continuous glucose monitors, or CGMs (the line), capture glucose curves that traditional finger prick tests (white circles) miss.

Now entire glucose curves are revealed and conveniently sent to your smartphone. It was a real game changer for people with diabetes, who rely on glucose measurements to dose their medication.

Soon after 23andMe launched the project, top athletes started to wear CGMs, too, using glucose measurements to optimize their athletic performance and endurance. And then a few scientific papers were published on studies using the devices that showed that nondiabetics could have highly dysregulated glucose levels, too.

When the Health Research & Development team announced a new study looking into food response in nondiabetics, I immediately asked to be a part of it. I was always on the lookout for something that could help me understand my own body. But I definitely did not expect what came of it.

A nurse came to our office to apply the device to the four of us who had volunteered. We waited for her in a glass-walled conference room; then we literally rolled up our sleeves. After wiping the back of my left upper arm with an alcohol swab, the nurse placed an applicator against my skin. I was told that a needle would go in and insert a tiny 3-millimeter-long fiber (an electrode) under my skin. Then the needle would come out, leaving the fiber in place and an adhesive transmitter on top of it. It would stay in for two weeks.

One, two . . . click! The monitor was in—and it was almost painless.

The sensor needed 60 minutes to start up, but then, with my phone handy, I could check my glucose levels at any time.* The numbers showed me how my body responded to what I ate (or didn't) and how I moved (or didn't). I was getting messages from the *inside*. Well, hello there, body!

When I felt great, I checked my glucose. When I felt terrible, I checked my glucose. When I worked out, when I woke up, when I went to sleep, I checked my glucose. My body was talking to me through the spikes and dips on my iPhone screen.

I ran my own experiments and took note of everything. My lab was my kitchen, my test subject was myself, and my hypothesis was that food and movement influence glucose through a set of rules that we could define.

Quite quickly, I started noticing strange patterns: Nachos on Monday, big spike. Nachos on Sunday, no spike. Beer, spike. Wine, no spike. M&Ms after lunch, no spike. M&Ms before dinner, spike. Tired in the afternoon: glucose had been high at lunch. Lots of energy all day: glucose was very steady. Big night out with friends: glucose roller coaster through the night. Stressful presentation at work: spike. Meditation: steady. Cappuccino when I was rested: no spike. Cappuccino when I was tired: spike. Bread: spike. Bread and butter: no spike.

Things got even more interesting as I linked my mental states to my glucose levels. My brain fog (which I had started experiencing since my accident) often correlated with a big spike, sleepiness with a big dip. Cravings correlated with a glucose roller coaster–spikes and

---

* Technically not in my blood but in the fluid between my cells. These are tightly correlated.

dips in quick succession. When I woke up feeling groggy, my glucose levels had been high throughout the night.

I sifted through the data, reran many experiments, and checked my hypothesis against published studies. To feel my best, it became clear that I had to avoid big spikes and dips in my glucose levels. And that was what I did: I learned how to flatten my glucose curves.

I was making transformative discoveries about my health. I cured my brain fog and curbed my cravings. When I woke up, I felt amazing. For the first time since my accident, I began to feel truly well again.

So I started telling my friends about it. That's how the Glucose Goddess movement began.

At first, I got a lot of blank stares. I showed my friends the studies and told them that they, too, should care about flattening their glucose curves. Crickets.

It became clear that I had to find a way of communicating those studies in an engaging way. I thought about using my own glucose data to illustrate the science. The problem was that at the outset, the insights from it were difficult to grasp.

A day's glucose data, right off the continuous glucose monitor.

To be able to make sense of it, I needed to "zoom in" to a specific time of day. But there was no way of doing so in the app the continuous glucose monitor came with. So I built software on my computer to do it myself.

I started keeping a diary of everything I ate. For each entry in my diary, I zoomed into four-hour windows. For instance, "5:56 p.m.— glass of orange juice". I looked at my glucose measurements starting one hour before I drank the juice and ending three hours later. Those gave me a convenient view of where my glucose levels were before I drank it, during, and after.

To make it easier on the eyes, I turned the dots into a line and filled in the spike.

And then, because science should be stylish, too, I simplified the axis and added an image of the food on the right. That was certainly more engaging.

My friends and family were fascinated by the graphs. They asked me to test more and more foods and share the results. And then they started getting their own continuous glucose monitors. They sent me

I zoomed into the four hours surrounding the time
I had drunk the orange juice, 5:56 p.m.

A finished graph with my homemade software.
Orange juice, and all other fruit juices, contain no fiber
and a lot of sugar. Drinking them leads to a glucose spike.

their data, and I aggregated it. One thing led to another, and after a while I didn't have enough time to keep up with the graph-making demand — so I built a phone app that automated it. My friends started using the app, friends of friends, too . . . it caught on like wildfire. Even friends without CGMs, buoyed by the evidence, started changing their eating habits.

And then, in April 2018, I started the @glucosegoddess Instagram account, and as the community grew and responded to my experiments and sent me results from their own, I became increasingly startled. Glucose, I realized, was associated with just about everything.

PART 1

~~~~~

What Is Glucose?

ENTER THE COCKPIT
Why Glucose Is So Important

Navigating our health sometimes feels like glancing into an airplane cockpit on the way to our seat. We see complicated stuff everywhere: screens, dials, flashing lights, knobs, switches, levers . . . buttons to the left, buttons to the right, buttons on the ceiling (no, but really, why do they have buttons on the *ceiling*?). We look away feeling grateful that the pilots know what they are doing. As passengers, all we care about is whether or not the plane stays in the air.

When it comes to our bodies, we are the clueless passengers, but—plot twist—we're also the pilots. And if we don't know how our bodies work, it's as if we're flying blind.

We know how we want to feel. We want to wake up with a smile, feeling energized and excited for the day. We want to have a skip in our step, feel pain free. We want to spend quality time with our loved ones, feeling positive and grateful. But it can be challenging to know how to get there. We're overwhelmed by all the buttons. What to do? Where to start?

We should start with glucose. Why? Because it's the lever in the cockpit with the biggest bang for its buck. It's the easiest to learn about (thanks to continuous glucose monitors), it affects how we feel *instantaneously* (because it influences our hunger and mood), and many things fall into place once we get it under control.

If our glucose levels are out of balance, dials flash and alarms go off. We put on weight, our hormones get out of whack, we feel tired, we crave sugar, our skin breaks out, our hearts suffer. We inch closer and closer to type 2 diabetes. If our body is the plane, the symptoms are the pitch, roll, and yaw of a machine out of control. And these strongly indicate that we need to rectify something to avoid a crash. To get back into ideal cruising mode, we need to flatten our glucose curves.

How do we move this lever? Very easily—with what's on our plate.

YES, THIS BOOK IS FOR YOU

A recent study showed that only 12 percent of Americans are metabolically healthy, which means that only 12 percent of Americans have a perfectly functioning body—including healthy glucose levels. Odds are that *you*, and nine out of the ten people closest to you, are on a glucose roller coaster without knowing it.

Here are some questions to ask yourself to find out if your glucose levels are dysregulated.

- Have you been told by a doctor that you need to lose weight?
- Are you trying to lose weight but finding it difficult?
- Is your waist size (or pant size) above 40 inches if you are a man or above 35 inches if you are a woman? (Waist size is better for predicting underlying disease than BMI is.)
- Do you have extreme hunger pangs during the day?
- Do you feel agitated or angry when you are hungry, aka *hangry*?
- Do you need to eat every few hours?

- Do you feel shaky, lightheaded, or dizzy if meals are delayed?
- Do you crave sweet things?
- Do you feel sleepy midmorning or midafternoon or are you tired all the time?
- Do you need caffeine to keep you going throughout the day?
- Do you have trouble sleeping or wake up with heart palpitations?
- Do you have energy crashes where you break out in a sweat or get nauseous?
- Do you suffer from acne, inflammation, or other skin conditions?
- Do you experience anxiety, depression, or mood disorders?
- Do you experience brain fog?
- Is your mood variable?
- Do you frequently get colds?
- Do you experience acid reflux or gastritis?
- Do you have hormonal imbalances, missed periods, PMS, infertility, or PCOS?
- Have you ever been told that your glucose levels are elevated?
- Do you have insulin resistance?
- Do you have prediabetes or type 2 diabetes?
- Do you have nonalcoholic fatty liver disease?
- Do you have heart disease?
- Do you have difficulty managing gestational diabetes?
- Do you have difficulty managing type 1 diabetes?

And most important: Do you think you could feel better than you currently do? If the answer is yes, keep reading.

WHAT THIS BOOK SAYS—AND WHAT IT DOESN'T

Before we dive in, it's important to know which conclusions *not* to draw from this book. Let me explain.

As a teenager, I went on a vegan diet. It was a *bad* vegan diet—instead of cooking nutrient-rich chickpea stews and loading up on crispy baked tofu and steamed edamame, I chose (vegan) Oreos and (vegan) pasta. All I ate was poor-quality, glucose-spiking food. My skin broke out in pimples, and I was constantly tired.

As a young adult I went on a keto diet. It was a *bad* keto diet. I had hoped to lose weight; instead I *gained* weight because in the process of removing all carbohydrates from my diet, all I ate was cheese. I stressed my hormonal system so much that my period stopped.

The more I've learned, the more I've realized that there is no benefit to extreme diets—especially because dogmas can easily be abused (there is very unhealthy vegan food, and there is very unhealthy keto food). The "diets" that work are the ones that flatten our glucose, fructose, and insulin curves. When vegan and keto are done well, they both do this. And when any diet is done well—meaning that it helps you reverse disease or lose excess weight—it's for that same reason. Really, we should be looking for sustainable lifestyles, not diets, and there is space on all our plates for a little bit of everything—including sugar. Knowing how glucose works has helped me understand that better than ever.

On the topic of being moderate, I want to note three important things to keep in mind as you read this book.

First, glucose isn't everything.

Some foods will keep your glucose levels completely steady but aren't great for your health. For instance, industrial processed oils and trans fats age, inflame, and hurt our organs, but they don't cause glucose spikes. Alcohol is another example—it doesn't spike our glucose levels, but that doesn't mean it's good for us, either.

Glucose isn't everything. There are other factors that determine our health: sleep, stress, exercise, emotional connection, medical care, and more. Beyond glucose, we should pay attention to fat, to fructose, and to insulin, too. I'll get to these later in this book. But both fructose and insulin levels are hard to monitor continuously. Glucose levels are the only measure we can track from the comfort of our couch, and the good news is that when we flatten our glucose curves, we also flatten our fructose and insulin curves. This is because fructose exists only hand in hand with glucose in foods and because insulin is released by our pancreas in response to glucose. When the numbers on insulin are available in the scientific studies (insulin is often measured continuously in clinical settings), I describe the effect of the hacks on them, too.

Second, context is key. My mother often sends me a photo of something she is debating buying at the supermarket. "Good or bad?" she texts. I always respond, "It depends—what would you eat instead?"

We can't say whether a food is good or bad in a vacuum—everything is relative. High-fiber pasta is "good" compared to regular pasta but "bad" compared to veggies. An oatmeal cookie is "bad" in relation to almonds but "good" in relation to a can of Coca-Cola. You see the conundrum. You cannot look at a single food's glucose curve and determine whether it is "good" or "bad." You must compare it to its alternative.

Finally, the recommendations here are always based on evidence. Every glucose graph in this book is here to illustrate scientific discoveries that I reference and cite. I do not draw generalized conclusions from a single person's glucose experiments or indeed from my own personal experiments. First, I do the research: I find scientific studies that explain how a certain habit flattens glucose curves—for example, a paper that finds that 10 minutes of moderate physical activity after a meal reduces the glucose spike of that meal. In these studies, the experiment has been run on a large group of people and the scientists have come to a generalized conclusion that statistically holds true. All I want to do is make a visual example of what they have found. So I pick a popular food that spikes glucose levels when eaten alone, such as a bag of chips. Then I eat the bag of chips on its own one morning, measure the resulting glucose curve, and do the same thing the next morning—but then go for a 10-minute walk. The second spike is smaller, just as the paper explains. That's what I show to people to illustrate that walking after any meal reduces the glucose spike of that meal. Sometimes it's not me but someone else from the Glucose Goddess community who contributes the illustrative test.

So if your body is a plane and you're both the pilot and the passenger, consider these three caveats your safety lesson. Now that you know that flattening your glucose curves is the place to start to get your body back to cruising altitude, buckle up: it's time to begin this journey by learning where glucose comes from.

MEET JERRY
How Plants Create Glucose

Plants don't get enough credit. To be fair, they rarely advertise their exploits. (They can't.) But if the cactus on your desk could speak, it would impress you with the tale of its ancestors: after all, they were the ones who invented the most important biological process on Earth—photosynthesis.

Millions of years ago, our planet was a barren rock of water and mud. Life consisted only of bacteria and wiggly worms in the oceans; no trees, no chirping birds, and certainly no mammals or humans.

Somewhere, in one of the corners of this blue planet, perhaps where South Africa is now, a magical thing happened. After millions of years of trial and error, a tiny sprout poked through the crust of the earth, opening one leaf and along with it a new chapter of the history of life.

Quite the feat. How did that sprout do it?

It was once common to assume that plants were "soil eaters": that they made themselves out of dirt. In the 1640s, a Flemish scientist by the name of Jan Baptist van Helmont set out to understand whether that was truly the case. He performed a five-year-long test known as the Willow Experiment, from which humanity learned two things: first, that van Helmont was very patient; second, that plants do *not* make themselves out of dirt.

Van Helmont planted a 5-pound baby willow tree in a large pot filled with 200 pounds of soil. For the next five years, he watered it and watched it grow. Then, after those five years had passed and the tree had grown, he took the tree out of the pot and weighed it again: it stood at 169 pounds—164 pounds heavier than it had been at the beginning. But most important, the weight of the *soil* in the pot remained virtually unchanged. That meant that the 164 pounds of tree had to have come from somewhere else.

So how do plants make their . . . plant stuff, if it isn't from soil? Back to the tiny sprout that just saw the light of day on Earth. Let's call him Jerry.

Jerry was the first to put together a very elegant solution: the ability to transform not soil but *air* into matter. Jerry combined carbon dioxide (from the air) and water (from the soil, but not actually soil), using the energy of the sun, to make a never-before-seen substance that he uses to construct every part of himself. This substance

5 years

The Willow Experiment
proved that plants aren't
made of dirt.

is what we now call *glucose*. Without glucose, there would be no plants and no life.

For hundreds of years after the Willow Experiment, hordes of researchers tried to understand how plants did what they did with the help of experiments involving candles, vacuum-sealed jars, and many different species of algae.

The three men who finally cracked it were American scientists by the names of Melvin Calvin, Andrew Benson, and James Bassham. For the discovery, Calvin was awarded the 1961 Nobel Prize in Chemistry. The process was baptized the "Calvin-Benson-Bassham Cycle." Since it's not the catchiest name, we commonly refer to it as *photosynthesis*: the process of turning carbon dioxide and water into glucose using the energy of the sun.

I'm a bit envious of the way plants do what they do. They don't have to spend any time at the grocery store. They create their own food. In human terms, it would be like being able to inhale molecules

Plants turn a sunny afternoon into glucose during photosynthesis and assemble glucose into various forms to grow. Here we see roots, leaves, and fruit.

from the air, sit in the sun, and create a creamy lentil soup inside our stomachs without needing to find it, cook it, or swallow it.

Once created, plants can either break down glucose to use as energy or keep it intact to use as a building block. And you couldn't dream of a better brick. It's so tiny and nimble that you could fit 500,000 molecules of it into the period at the end of this sentence. It can be used to make the plant's rigid trunk, flexible leaves, spindly roots, or juicy fruit. Just as diamonds or pencil lead can be made from the exact same atom (carbon), plants can make many different things out of glucose.

STRONG STARCH

Among the things plants can make from glucose is *starch*.

A living plant needs a supply of energy at all times. However, when it's not sunny out, either because it's cloudy or because it's dark, photosynthesis cannot take place and provide the plant with the glucose it needs to survive. In order to solve this problem, plants make extra glucose during the day and pack it away into reserves for later use.

The thing is, storing glucose isn't easy. Glucose's natural tendency is to dissolve into everything around it, like children let loose onto a playground at recess. Kids race and dash in random directions, generally uncontrollably and unpredictably, but can be rounded up by their teacher and sit (mostly) quietly behind their desks when class begins again. Similarly, plants have a solution to round up glucose. They enlist tiny helpers called *enzymes*—teacher's aides, if you will—that grab glucose molecules by the hand and attach them to each other: left hand with right hand, left hand with right hand, hundreds and thousands of times over. The result is a long chain of glucose, no longer racing and dashing in random directions.

This form of glucose is called *starch*. It can be stored in small amounts throughout the plant, but mostly in its roots.

glucose   starch

**Plants assemble glucose into long chains
called *starch* in order to store it.**

Beets, potatoes, carrots, celeriac, parsnips, turnips, jicama, and yams are all roots, and all contain starch. Seeds also contain starch, which provides the necessary energy to help them grow into a plant. Rice, oatmeal, corn, wheat, barley, beans, peas, lentils, soybeans, and chickpeas are all seeds, and all of them contain starch, too.

Discipline reins in starch in that classroom—so much so that "starch" comes from the Germanic word that means "strong."

Starch really is strong, but that doesn't mean it's inflexible. It can be taken apart with the right tool. Whenever plants need

**Root vegetables and seeds
are packed with starch.**

glucose, they use an enzyme called alpha-amylase that heads to the roots and frees some glucose molecules from their starch chains. *Snap*—glucose is let loose, ready to be used as energy or as a building block.

FIERCE FIBER

Another enzyme (there are a number of them) can be called on to perform a different task: to create *fiber*. Instead of attaching glucose molecules hand to hand to make starch, this enzyme connects glucose molecules hand to foot, and the resulting chain is called *fiber*. This substance is as important as grout between the bricks of a house. It's what allows plants to grow tall without falling over. It's most commonly found in trunks, branches, flowers, and leaves, but there is fiber in roots and fruit as well.

Humans found a practical purpose for fiber: it was harvested and processed to create paper, from Egyptian papyruses onward. Today, it's extracted from tree trunks, polymerized, and turned into sheets

Trunks, branches, and leaves contain the most fiber.

and reams of paper. If you're reading these words in a physical book, you're reading a book about glucose printed on glucose.

FLIRTY FRUIT

If you were to lick glucose, it would taste sweet. But plants also transform some of their glucose into an *extra-sweet* molecule called *fructose*, which is about 2.3 times as sweet as glucose.

Plants concentrate fructose into fruit—apples, cherries, kiwis, and more—that they dangle from their branches. The purpose of fructose is to make fruit taste irresistible to animals. Why do plants want their fruit to be irresistible? Because they hide their seeds in them. It's key to propagation: plants hope that animals will eat their fruit and their seeds will go unnoticed until they come out their eater's other end. That's how seeds spread far and wide, thereby ensuring plants' survival.

Most of plants' fructose is used in this way, but some, with the help of another enzyme, links up, for a time, with glucose. The result is a molecule called *sucrose*. Sucrose exists to help plants compress energy even further (a sucrose molecule is slightly smaller than a

Fruits are full of fructose.

glucose and fructose molecule side by side, which allows plants to store more energy in a tighter space). For plants, sucrose is an ingenious temporary storage solution, but for us, it has a huge significance. We use it every day, under a different name: table sugar.

Starch, fiber, fructose, and sucrose—the various forms glucose can take—exist thanks to photosynthesis. And this, Jerry's elegant solution, paved the way for the rest of life on this planet.

A FAMILY AFFAIR
How Glucose Gets into the Bloodstream

The glucose-burning system that plants invented became vital to all living things, from dinosaurs to dolphins to mice. Four hundred forty-nine million years after the first plant appeared, humans arrived—and they burned glucose, too.

Your cells, like all animal and plant cells, need energy to stay alive—and glucose is their *prioritized* energy source. Each of our cells uses glucose for energy according to its specific function. Your heart cells use it to contract, your brain cells to fire neurons, your ear cells to hear, your eye cells to see, your stomach cells to digest, your skin cells to repair cuts, your red blood cells to bring oxygen to your feet so you can dance all night long.

Every *second*, your body burns 8 billion billion molecules of glucose. To put that into perspective, if each glucose molecule were a grain of sand, you'd burn every single grain of sand on all the beaches of the earth *every ten minutes*.

Suffice it to say, humans need a tremendous amount of fuel.

There is just one tiny hiccup: humans aren't plants. Even with the very best of intentions, we can't make glucose from the air and the sun. (I tried to photosynthesize at the beach once—to no avail.)

The most common way (but not the only way) for us to get the glucose we need is by eating it.

Starch

When I was 11 years old, we conducted an experiment in biology class that I remember to this day. We sat down for second period, and each student was handed a slice of white bread.

As we looked around perplexed, our teacher broke the news: we were to put the whole slice in our mouth and chew it—fighting the urge to swallow—for a full minute. It was an odd request but arguably more fun than our usual class activities, so off we went.

About 30 chews in, something surprising happened: the taste of the bread started shifting—it began to taste sweet!

Starch was turning into glucose in my mouth.

A slice of bread is made, for the most part, from flour. Flour is made by grinding wheat kernels, and wheat kernels, as you know, are filled with starch. Any food made from flour contains starch. Pie crust, cookies, pastries, pasta—all are composed of flour, so all are composed of starch. When we eat, we break starch down into glucose, using the same enzyme that plants use to do this task: alpha-amylase.

Starch is turned into glucose extremely quickly in our body. In general, the process happens mostly in our gut, where it goes unnoticed. The alpha-amylase enzymes snap the bonds of the chain, and glucose molecules are freed. There they are, running around in the playground once again.

The enzymes that do this vital work also exist in our saliva. When we chew starch long enough, we give the enzymes the time they need to begin their work. That process begins in our mouth, and we can taste it. Hence the power of this experiment.

Fruit

Fruit, in contrast, tastes sweet from the get-go. This is because it already contains unchained glucose molecules, which taste sweet, as well as fructose, which tastes even sweeter, and their combined form, sucrose, which is sweeter than glucose but not as sweet as fructose.

Glucose from fruit is ready to be used and does not need to be snapped. Sucrose does need to be snapped, and there's an enzyme that separates it into glucose and fructose molecules, but this does not take long—it happens in a nanosecond.

Fructose is a little more complicated. After we eat it, a portion of it is turned back into glucose in our small intestine. The remainder of it stays in fructose form. Both permeate the lining of our gut to enter our bloodstream. I'll explain what happens next later in this book, but what I want you to remember now is that although glucose is needed to fuel your body's systems, fructose isn't. We eat a lot of unnecessary fructose in our diet nowadays, because we eat a lot more sucrose (which, as a reminder, is half glucose, half fructose).

What about fiber? Well, it has a special fate.

Fiber

Enzymes work to snap the bonds of starch and sucrose, but there is no enzyme that can snap the bonds of fiber. It doesn't get turned back into glucose. This is why when we eat fiber, it remains fiber. It travels from our stomach to our small and large intestines. And this is a good thing. Though it doesn't turn back into glucose and therefore can't provide energy to our cells, fiber is an essential part of our diet and plays a very important role in aiding digestion, maintaining healthy bowel movements, keeping our microbiome healthy, and more.

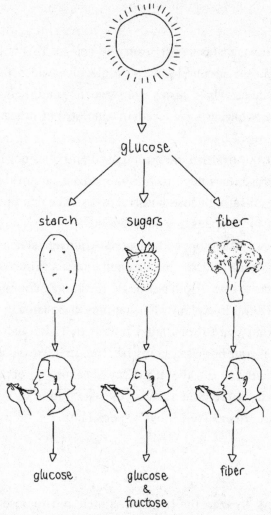

glucose

starch   sugars   fiber

glucose   glucose   fiber
              &
              fructose

Any part of a plant we eat turns back into glucose (and fructose)
as we digest it, except for fiber, which passes right through us.

ONE PARENT, FOUR SIBLINGS

Starch, fiber, fructose, and sucrose are like four siblings with different personalities. They're all related, because they have the same
parent, glucose—no matter how much they argue about who bor-
rowed whose clothes.

It would almost make sense to give them a family name.

In 1969, a cohort of scientists wrote a 20-page-long document titled "Tentative Rules for Carbohydrate Nomenclature, Part I, 1969" and presented it to the scientific community.

After that paper, it was accepted that the name for this family would be "carbohydrates." Why carbohydrates? Because it refers to things that were made by joining carbon (carbo) and water (hydrate), which is what happens during photosynthesis.

You may have heard of this family under its popular nickname, *carbs*.

Carbohydrates = Starch and Fiber and Sugars (glucose, fructose, sucrose)

You'll notice that within the carbohydrate family (which includes starch, fiber, glucose, fructose, and sucrose), scientists decided to make a subgroup for the smallest molecules: glucose, fructose, and sucrose. This subgroup is called *sugars*. The scientific word *sugars* is not the same as our common table sugar, even though the *sugars* group does include the molecule that constitutes table sugar, sucrose. That's scientific nomenclature for you.

Members of the carbohydrate family exist in various proportions in a plant. For example, broccoli contains a lot of fiber and some starch, potatoes contain a lot of starch and some fiber, and peaches contain mostly sugars and some fiber (you'll notice that there is at least *some* fiber in every plant).

But a bit confusingly, when people talk about nutrition, they often say "carbohydrates" or "carbs" to describe only starch and sugars. They don't include fiber, because it isn't absorbed into our bloodstream as its siblings are. You might hear something such as "Broccoli has few carbs but a lot of fiber." According to the scientific nomenclature, the correct thing to say would be "Broccoli contains a lot of carbs, most of which are fiber."

I will stick to convention here, because it's most likely what you'll hear from those around you. (But as always, I wanted you to understand the science!) When I say "carbohydrates" or "carbs," I'll be talking about starchy foods (potatoes, pasta, rice, bread, and so on) and sugary foods (fruit, pies, cakes, and more) but not about vegetables, because they contain mostly fiber and very little starch. And I will say "sugar" when I'm referring to table sugar, as most of us do.

WHAT IF THERE WAS NO GLUCOSE IN OUR DIET?

Since glucose is so important to life, you may wonder how some carnivorous animals survive. After all, many animals don't eat plants (for instance dolphins, which feast on fish, squid, and jellyfish), and some humans evolved in areas without a fruit or vegetable in sight, as in the freezing Russian plains, so they didn't eat plants, either.

Well, because glucose is so important to our cells, if we can't find any to eat, our body can *make it from within*. That's right, we don't photosynthesize and make glucose out of air, water, and sunlight, but we can make glucose from the food we eat—from fat or protein. Our liver, through a process called *gluconeogenesis*, performs this process.

What's more, our bodies adapt even further: when glucose is limited, many cells in our body can, when needed, switch to using fat for fuel instead. This is called *metabolic flexibility*. (The only cells that always rely on glucose are red blood cells.)

Indeed, some diets such as Atkins and keto deliberately restrict the consumption of carbohydrates in order to keep a person's glucose levels extremely low and thus push the body into burning fat for fuel. This is called *nutritional ketosis* and is metabolic flexibility in action.

So, sure, carbohydrates aren't biologically *necessary* (we don't need to eat sugar to live), but they are a quick source of energy and a delicious part of our diet, and they have been consumed for millions of years. Scientists know that humans' prehistoric diet included both animals and plants: when plants were available, humans consumed them. What they ate depended on where they lived. They adapted to the unique food supply around them. And our food supply today looks quite different from what nature had planned.

SEEKING PLEASURE
Why We Eat More Glucose than Before

Nature intended us to consume glucose in a specific way: in plants. Wherever there was starch or sugar, there was fiber as well. This is important, because the fiber helped to slow our body's absorption of glucose. You'll learn how to use this information to your advantage in part 3.

Today, however, the vast majority of supermarket shelves are packed with products that contain mostly starch and sugar. From white bread to ice cream, candy, fruit juices, and sweetened yogurts, fiber is nowhere to be seen. And this is on purpose: fiber is often removed in the creation of processed foods, because its presence is problematic if you're trying to preserve things for a long time.

Let me explain—and I have to admit, strawberries were harmed in the making of this example. Place a fresh strawberry in the freezer overnight. The next morning, take it out to thaw on a plate. If you try to eat it, it will be mushy. Why? Because the fiber was broken into smaller bits by the freezing and thawing process. The fiber is still there (and still has health benefits), but the texture is not the same.

**A fresh strawberry; then what it looks like
after it is frozen overnight and thawed.**

Fiber is often removed from processed foods so that they can be frozen, thawed, and last on shelves for years without losing their texture. Take, for example, white flour: fiber is found in the germ and bran (outer husk) of the wheat kernel, so the bran is stripped away during milling.

Something else is done to foods to turn them into successful supermarket products: their sweetness is increased. The basis of food processing is to first strip away the fiber, then concentrate the starch and sugars.

Indeed, when we humans find something good, we tend to take it to the extreme. The smell of fresh roses pleases our senses, so

**When the starchy parts of plants are processed to make supermarket
goods, they are stripped of their fiber. Fiber-packed seeds and roots
are turned into starchy bread or chips (and sugar is usually added).**

thousands of tons of rose petals are distilled and concentrated into essential oil, bottled, and made available anywhere, anytime, by the perfumery industry. Similarly, the food industry wanted to distill and concentrate nature's most sought-after taste: sweetness.

You may wonder: Why do we like sweetness so much? It's because in Stone Age times the taste of sweetness signaled foods that were both safe (there are no foods that are both sweet and poisonous) *and* packed with energy. In a time when food wasn't easy to find, it was an advantage to eat all the fruit before anyone else could, so we evolved to feel pleasure when we tasted something sweet.

When we do, a hit of a chemical called dopamine floods our brain. This is the same chemical that is released when we have sex, play video games, scroll social media or, with more dangerous consequences, drink alcohol, smoke cigarettes, or use illegal drugs. And we can never get enough of it.

In a 2016 study, mice were given a lever with which they could activate their own dopamine neurons (thanks to a special optical sensor). The researchers saw a peculiar behavior: if they left the mice to their own devices, the mice spent all their time pressing the lever to activate their dopamine neurons, over and over. They stopped eating and drinking—to the point where eventually the researchers had to end the experiment because otherwise, the mice were going to die. The mice's dopamine obsession had made them forget their basic needs. This is all to say that animals, including humans, *really* like dopamine. And eating sweet foods is an easy way to get a hit.

Plants have been concentrating glucose, fructose, and sucrose in their fruit forever, but a few millennia ago humans began to do the same: we started breeding plants so that, among other reasons, their fruit would taste even sweeter.

And then, by boiling sugarcane and crystallizing its juice, humans created table sugar—100 percent sucrose. This new product became

Ancestral bananas are as nature intended them to be:
full of fiber, with a small amount of sugar.
The twenty-first-century banana (bottom image)
is the result of many generations of breeding
to reduce the fiber and increase the sugar.

On the left, a peach as it was six thousand years ago. On
the right, a twenty-first-century peach. The fruits we eat
today are sweeter than they were thousands of years ago.

very popular in the eighteenth century. As the demand grew, so did
the horrors of slavery: millions of slaves were taken to humid parts of
the world to farm sugarcane and produce table sugar.

Sugar sources changed over time—we now extract sucrose
from beets and corn, too—but regardless of which plant is used, the

Fruit, such as cherries, and candy, such as jelly beans, both contain sugar. But jelly beans contain a superconcentrated amount of it.

resulting sucrose added to processed foods is the chemical copy of the one found in fruit. What's different is its concentration.

Sugar has become ever more concentrated and available: we have gone from eating in-season foraged fibrous fruit in prehistoric times to eating minuscule quantities of sucrose in the 1800s (you'd have been lucky if you came across a single candy bar in your entire life) to eating more than *94 pounds* of the stuff per year today.

We keep eating more of it because it's hard for our brain to curb its cravings for things that taste like fruit. Sweetness and dopamine feel forever rewarding.

As the mice experiment shows, it's important to understand that the inclination to reach for a candy bar isn't our fault. It's not a

Even tomatoes have been turned into a sweeter version of themselves: ketchup.

willpower issue—far from it. Deep, old evolutionary programming tells us that eating Skittles is a good move.

Sheryl Crow sings that if something makes you happy *"it can't be that bad."* We need glucose to live, and it gives us pleasure. So it's fair to wonder: What's the big deal if we eat more?

In some cases, more isn't necessarily better. Give a plant too much water, and it will drown; give humans too much oxygen, and they pass out. Similarly, there is an amount of glucose that is *just right* for us: just enough for us to feel great, jump around, go to work, hang out with other humans, live, laugh, and love. But we can have too much glucose. And too much glucose hurts us, often without our realizing it.

UNDERNEATH OUR SKIN
Discovering Glucose Spikes

A long time ago, way before I knew about glucose, I ate a Nutella crepe every morning before school. I would wake up 20 minutes before I had to leave the house, pull on jeans and a T-shirt, forget to brush my hair (sorry, Mom), head to the kitchen, grab crepe mix from the fridge, place a slab of butter on a hot pan, pour the mix onto it, *swish swish*, flip it, plate it, lather it with Nutella, fold it, and eat it.

I would say goodbye to my mom, who was enjoying her own breakfast: a bowl of Special K and milk sprinkled with table sugar, and a glass of orange juice.

Millions of people were eating a similar breakfast. On the table was a display of some pretty cool technology. For me: wheat milled and turned into flour; sucrose, hazelnuts, palm oil, and cocoa blended into a spread. For my mom: grains of corn popped and turned into flakes; beets squished and pureed and dried into sucrose; and oranges juiced into a liquid consisting mostly of glucose and fructose.

All that concentrated sugar tasted very sweet. Our tongues whole-tonguedly approved of the party.

The starch and sugar turned into glucose after we swallowed them; they landed in our stomach, then entered our small intestine. There, the glucose disappeared through the lining of our gut and moved into our bloodstream. From our capillaries—tiny blood vessels—it moved to larger and larger vessels, just like taking the on-ramp to a freeway.

When doctors measure the amount of glucose in our body, they often draw our blood and assess its concentration there. But glucose doesn't just stay in our blood. It seeps into every part of us, and it can be measured anywhere.

That's why with a continuous glucose monitor (CGM), I can measure the amount of glucose throughout my body without a blood draw: the CGM senses the concentration of glucose between the fat cells on the back of my arm.

To quantify the concentration of glucose, we use milligrams per deciliter, also written mg/dL. Other countries use millimoles per liter (mmol/L). Whatever unit is used, they refer to the same thing: how much glucose is freely roaming in the body.

The American Diabetes Association (ADA) states that a baseline concentration (also known as your *fasting level*, that is, your glucose level first thing in the morning before eating) between 60 and 100 mg/dL is "normal"; that between 100 and 126 mg/dL indicates prediabetes; and anything above 126 mg/dL indicates diabetes.

But what the ADA describes as "normal" may not actually be optimal. Early studies showed that the *thriving* range for fasting glucose may be between 72 and 85 mg/dL. That's because there is more likelihood of developing health problems from 85 mg/dL and up.

Furthermore, though our fasting level gives us information on whether we are at risk for being diagnosed with diabetes or not, it isn't the only thing to consider. Even if our fasting level is "optimal," we may still experience *glucose spikes* on a daily basis. Spikes are rapid increases and drops in glucose concentration after we eat, and they are harmful. I'll explain why in the next chapter.

The ADA states that our glucose levels shouldn't increase above 140 mg/dL after eating. But again, that's "normal," not optimal. Studies in nondiabetics give more precise information: we should strive to avoid increasing our glucose levels by more than 30 mg/dL after eating. So in this book I will define a *glucose spike* as an increase in glucose in our body of more than 30 mg/dL after eating.

The goal is to avoid spikes, whatever your fasting level is, because it's the *variability* caused by spikes that is most problematic. It's *years* of repeated daily spikes that slowly increase our fasting glucose level, a pattern we discover only once that level is classified as prediabetic. By then, the damage has already started.

Every morning, my mom's breakfast led to a massive glucose spike of 80 mg/dL, taking her fasting level of 100 mg/dL all the way up to 180 mg/dL! That increase was well above the 30 mg/dL measure of a spike and even well above the 140 mg/dL ADA cutoff for a "normal" spike after a meal.

The traditional cereal breakfast, thought of as healthy, makes our glucose spike way beyond the healthy range and then come crashing down just as quickly.

On the top, a week's glucose curves with many spikes;
on the bottom, a week with fewer spikes.

Remember that the measurements of the concentration of glucose in your body over time, when plotted, create a *glucose curve*. For example, if I look at my glucose levels for the past week, my curve will be variable if I experienced many spikes or flat if I experienced fewer spikes.

In this book, I advise you to flatten your glucose curves, which means zooming out and seeing fewer and smaller spikes over time. Another way to describe flattening your glucose curves is *reducing glycemic variability*. The smaller your glycemic variability, the better your health will be.

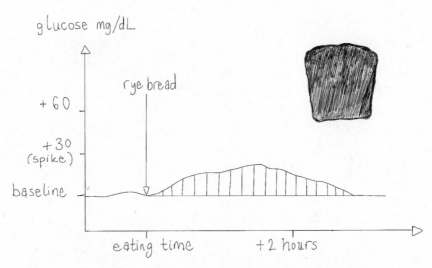

**When comparing two curves, you don't need to do any math.
The one with the taller spike, i.e., the most variability
(the rice cake one), is worse for your health.**

SOME SPIKES ARE WORSE THAN OTHERS

The two glucose spikes charted below look exactly the same. But one was more harmful to my body than the other. Can you guess which one?

A glucose spike from a sweet food (cupcake) is worse for our health than a glucose spike from a starchy food (rice). The reason has nothing to do with the glucose measured, though; it has to do with a molecule that's not visible.

A sweet food contains table sugar, or sucrose—that compound made up of glucose and fructose. A starchy food doesn't. Whenever we see a glucose spike from a sweet food, there is a corresponding fructose spike that unfortunately we can't see. Continuous glucose monitors can detect only glucose, not fructose, and continuous fructose monitors don't exist yet.

Until they do, remember that if the food you ate was sweet and it created a glucose spike, it also created an invisible fructose spike, and that's what makes a sweet spike more harmful than a starchy spike.

Now it's time to get to the *why*: Why exactly are glucose spikes bad for us, and why are fructose spikes worse? What do they do inside our body? Put your glasses on, grab a beverage, and get comfortable. By the end of part 2 you'll have learned your body's language.

PART 2

~~~~~~

Why Are Glucose Spikes Harmful?

TRAINS, TOAST, AND TETRIS

The Three Things that Happen in Our Body When We Spike

E ach of us is made up of more than 30 trillion cells. When we spike, they all feel it.

   Glucose's primary biological purpose once it enters a cell is to be turned into energy. The powerhouses responsible for this are microscopic organelles called *mitochondria*. Using glucose (and oxygen from the air we breathe), they create the chemical version of electricity to give each cell the power to do whatever it needs to. As glucose floods into our cells, it heads straight to the mitochondria to undergo its transformation.

WHY THE TRAIN STOPS: FREE RADICALS AND OXIDATIVE STRESS

To understand how mitochondria respond to a glucose spike coming their way, imagine this: your grandfather, finally retiring after a long career, is able to fulfill his dream of working on a steam train.

Everyone in the family thinks he's crazy for doing it, but he doesn't care. After some training, he enlists as a stoker in a train's engine room: his job is to shovel coal onto the fire to generate the steam that pushes the pistons and makes the wheels of the train turn. He's the mitochondria of the train, if you will.

Periodically throughout the day, as the train speeds along the tracks, coal is delivered to your grandfather. He places it by the furnace and shovels it into the flames at a steady pace to fuel the process that moves the train. The raw material is converted to energy. And when the stock is used up, another batch is promptly supplied.

Just like the train, our cells hum along smoothly when the amount of energy that is provided matches up with the amount of energy needed to function.

Now it's the second day of your grandfather's new job. A few minutes after the first delivery of coal, he gets a surprising knock on the door. More coal. He thinks, *Well, it's a bit early, but that way I'll have some extra.* He sets it aside next to the furnace. A few minutes later, another knock. More coal. And another. The knocks keep coming, and the coal keeps being delivered. "I don't need all of this!" he says. But he's told that it's his job to burn it, and he's given no other explanation.

All day long, delivery after delivery, unnecessary coal is stuffed into his cabin. The coal being delivered far exceeds what is needed. Your grandfather can't burn the coal more quickly, so piles build up around him.

In a short while, there's coal everywhere, stacked to the ceiling. He can barely move. He can't shovel any more coal onto the fire because there is so much in the way. The train stops, and people get angry. At the end of the day, he quits, his dream sabotaged.

Mitochondria feel the same way when we give them more glucose than they need. They can burn only as much glucose as the cell needs for energy, not more. When we spike, we deliver glucose to our

**A healthy cell contains
thousands of functioning
mitochondria, among
many other components.**

cells *too quickly*. The speed — or *velocity* — at which it is delivered is
the issue. Too much at once, and problems pile up.

According to the latest scientific theory, the Allostatic Load
Model, when our mitochondria are drowning in unnecessary glucose,
tiny molecules with large consequences are released: *free radicals*.
(And some glucose is converted to fat; more on that shortly.) When
free radicals appear because of a spike, they set off a dangerous chain
reaction.

Free radicals are a big deal because anything they touch, they
damage. They randomly snap and modify our genetic code (our
DNA), creating mutations that activate harmful genes and can lead
to the development of cancer. They poke holes in the membranes
of our cells, turning a normally functioning cell into a malfunction-
ing one.

Under normal circumstances, we live with a moderate amount
of free radicals, and we can handle them — but with repeated spikes,
the quantity produced becomes unmanageable. When there are too

Cell attacked by free radicals

Normal cell

cell with oxidative stress

many free radicals to be neutralized, our body is said to be in a state of *oxidative stress.*

Oxidative stress is a driver of heart disease, type 2 diabetes, cognitive decline, and general aging. And fructose increases oxidative stress even more than glucose alone. That's one of the reasons that sweet foods (which contain fructose) are worse than starchy foods (which don't). Too much fat can also increase oxidative stress.

Over decades cells become ravaged. Because they're stuffed, crowded, and overwhelmed, our mitochondria can't convert glucose to energy efficiently. The cells starve, which leads to organ dysfunction. We feel this as humans: even though we're fueling up by eating, we suffer from lassitude; it's hard to get up in the morning, and we have no energy throughout the day. We're *tired.* Do you know the feeling? I sure did.

That feeling is compounded by a second process that's set off when we experience a glucose spike.

WHY YOU ARE TOASTING: GLYCATION AND INFLAMMATION

This may come as a surprise to you, but you are currently *cooking*. More specifically, you are *browning*, just like a slice of bread in the toaster.

Inside our body, from the moment we are born, things literally brown, albeit very slowly. When scientists look at the rib cage cartilage of babies, it's white. Once a human reaches 90 years old, that same cartilage is brown.

In 1912, a French chemist by the name of Louis-Camille Maillard described and gave his name to this phenomenon, now known as the Maillard reaction. He discovered that *browning* happens when a glucose molecule bumps into another type of molecule. That causes a reaction. The second molecule is then said to be "glycated." When a molecule is glycated, it's damaged.

This process is a normal and inevitable part of life, and it's why we age, why our organs slowly deteriorate, and why we eventually die. We can't stop this process, but we can slow it down or speed it up.

When we toast bread, we make it brown.
Our insides are browning just like this.

The more glucose we deliver to our body, the more often glycation happens. Once a molecule is glycated, it's damaged forever—which is why you can't untoast a piece of toast. The long-term consequences of glycated molecules range from wrinkles and cataracts to heart disease and Alzheimer's disease. Since browning is aging and aging is browning, slowing down the browning reaction in your body leads to a longer life.

Fructose molecules glycate things *10 times as fast as glucose*, generating that much more damage. Again, this is another reason why spikes from sugary foods such as cookies (which contain fructose) make us age faster than do spikes from starchy foods such as pasta (which doesn't).

Glucose levels and glycation are so connected that a very common test to measure the level of glucose in our body actually measures glycation. The hemoglobin A1c (HbA1c) test (well known among diabetics) measures how many red blood cell proteins have been glycated by glucose over the past two to three months. The higher your HbA1c level, the more often the Maillard reaction is happening inside your body, the more glucose is circulating, and the faster you are aging.

The combination of too many free radicals, oxidative stress, and glycation leads to a generalized state of *inflammation* in the body. Inflammation is a protective measure; it's the result of the body trying to defend against invaders. But chronic inflammation is harmful because it turns against our own body. From the outside, you might see redness and swelling, and on the inside, tissues and organs are slowly getting damaged.

Inflammation can also be driven up by alcohol, smoking, stress, leaky gut syndrome, and substances released by body fat. Chronic inflammation is the source of most chronic illnesses, such as stroke, chronic respiratory diseases, heart disorders, liver disease, obesity, and diabetes. The World Health Organization calls inflammation-based diseases "the greatest threat to human health." Worldwide, three out of five people will die of an inflammation-based disease.

The good news is, a diet that reduces glucose spikes decreases inflammation and along with it your risk of contracting any of these inflammation-based diseases.

The third and final process we are going to dive into might be the most surprising. It's actually a defense mechanism that our body uses to defend against spikes—but it has its own consequences.

PLAYING TETRIS TO SURVIVE: INSULIN AND FAT GAIN

It's essential to our survival to get excess glucose out of circulation as quickly as possible, to reduce free radical formation and glycation. So our body, working without our even knowing it, has a plan: it starts playing a kind of Tetris.

In Tetris, players arrange blocks into rows to clear them before they accumulate. It's eerily similar to what happens in our body: as too much glucose enters, our body does its best to stash it away.

Here's how it works.

When our glucose levels increase, our pancreas becomes the *chef d'orchestre* of Tetris.

One of the pancreas's main functions is to send a hormone called

Tetris? No—the clearing of a glucose spike.

insulin into the body. Insulin's sole purpose is to stash excess glucose in storage units throughout the body, to keep it out of circulation and protect us from damage. Without insulin, we would die; people without the ability to make it—who have type 1 diabetes—must inject insulin to make up for what the pancreas can't produce.

Insulin stashes excess glucose in several storage units. Enter storage unit number one: the *liver*. The liver is a very convenient storage unit, because all the blood that comes from the gut carrying new glucose from digestion has to go through the liver.

Our liver turns glucose into a new form, called glycogen. It's equivalent to how plants turn glucose into starch. Glycogen is actually the cousin of starch—it's composed of many glucose molecules attached hand to hand. If excess glucose stayed in its original form, it would cause oxidative stress and glycation. Once transformed, it does no damage.

The liver can hold about 100 grams of glucose in glycogen form (the amount of glucose in two large McDonald's fries). That's half of the 200 grams of glucose that our body needs for energy per day.

The second storage unit is our *muscles*. Our muscles are effective storage units because we have so many of them. The muscles of a typical 150-pound adult can hold about 400 grams of glucose as glycogen, or the amount of glucose in seven large McDonald's fries.

The liver and muscles are efficient, but we tend to eat much more glucose than we need, so those storage units get full rather quickly. Fairly soon, if we didn't have another storage unit for extra glucose, our body would lose its game of Tetris.

Which part of our body can we grow very easily, without much effort and just by sitting on our couch? Introducing our fat reserves.

Once insulin has stored all the glucose it can in our liver and muscles, any glucose beyond that is turned into fat and stored in our fat reserves. And that's one of the ways we put on weight.

And then some. Because it's not just glucose that our body has to deal with, it must also dispose of fructose. And unfortunately,

Glucose
is stored as...

Fructose
is stored as...

Glycogen
(in liver and muscles)

Fat
(in fat cells)

Fat
(in fat cells)

**Humans store extra glucose as glycogen and fat.
Extra fructose just turns into fat.**

fructose cannot be turned into glycogen and stored in the liver and the muscles. The only thing that fructose can be stored as is fat.

The fat our body creates from fructose has a few unfortunate destinies: first, it accumulates in the liver and drives the development of nonalcoholic fatty liver disease. Second, it fills up fat cells in our hips, thighs, and face and between our organs, and we gain weight. Finally, it enters the bloodstream and contributes to an increased risk of heart disease. (You may have heard of it as low-density lipoprotein [LDL] or "bad" cholesterol.)

This is another reason why, if two foods have the same amount of calories, I'd recommend that you skip the sweet food (which contains fructose) in favor of a savory food (which doesn't). The absence of fructose means that fewer molecules end up as fat.

Ironically, processed foods that are "fat free" often contain a lot of sucrose, so the fructose in it is turned into fat after we digest it. More on this in part 3.

Many of us have complicated feelings about fat, but it's actually very useful: your body uses its fat reserves to provide storage space for the excess glucose and fructose floating around in your

About **60** minutes after a meal, our glucose concentration reaches
its maximum and then starts coming down as insulin arrives and
ushers the glucose molecules away into our liver, muscles, and fat cells.

bloodstream. We shouldn't be mad at our body for putting on fat; instead, we should thank it for trying to protect us from oxidative stress, glycation, and inflammation. The more you're able to grow the number and size of your fat cells (which is usually a function of genetics), the longer you'll be protected against excess glucose and fructose (but the more weight you will put on).

Which brings me back to insulin. Insulin, as I've explained, is vital to this process, as it helps stash excess glucose in those three "storage lockers." And in the short term it's helpful. But the more glucose spikes we experience, the more insulin is released in our bodies. In the long term, chronically elevated levels of insulin bring problems of their own. Too much insulin is the root cause of obesity, type 2 diabetes, polycystic ovarian syndrome (PCOS), and more. One of the most important things that happens when we flatten our glucose curves is that we automatically flatten our insulin curves as well.

Back to those complicated feelings about fat. It's useful, but if you're trying to shed pounds, it's important to understand what's happening in your body on a cellular level and how insulin makes things tricky. When we say "I want to lose weight," what we're actually saying is "I want to empty my fat cells of the fat they contain so that they deflate, like balloons, reduce in size, and, with them, my waist size." To do so, we need to be in "fat-burning" mode.

Just as Jerry could tap into his starch reserves at night, our body can call on glycogen in our liver and muscles to turn back into glucose whenever the thousands of mitochondria in each cell need it. Then, when our glycogen reserves begin to diminish, our body draws on the fat in our fat reserves for energy—we're in fat-burning mode—and we lose weight.

But this happens only when our insulin levels are low. If there is insulin present, our body is prevented from burning fat: insulin makes the route to our fat cells a one-way street: things can go in, but nothing can come out. We're not able to burn any existing reserves until our insulin levels start coming back down about two hours after the spike.

But if our glucose levels, and therefore our insulin levels, are steady, we shed pounds. In a 2021 study of 5,600 people, Canadian scientists showed that weight loss is always preceded by insulin decrease.

Excess glucose in our body and the spikes and dips it causes change us on a cellular level. Weight gain is just one of the symptoms we can see; there are many more. But for each, flattening our glucose curves can bring relief.

FROM HEAD TO TOE
How Spikes Make Us Sick

Early on, I had a profound realization that kick-started my research into glucose: *how I feel right now* is intimately linked to the spikes and dips of my glucose curve.

One day at work, around 11 a.m., I had grown so sleepy that I could barely move my fingers to click my mouse. Focusing on the task at hand was impossible. So, with a lot of effort, I stood up, walked to the office kitchen, and poured myself a large black coffee. I drank the whole cup—and still I was exhausted. I checked my glucose levels: they had been on a steep downward slope since a big spike after a breakfast made of a salt and chocolate chip cookie and a cappuccino with skim milk. I was tired because I was on a glucose roller coaster.

As I've discovered more about glucose, I've learned that there is a wide array of unwelcome short-term symptoms associated with spikes and dips, and they vary from person to person. For some, they're dizziness, nausea, heart palpitations, sweats, food cravings, and stress; for others, like me, they're exhaustion and brain fog. And

The big drop in glucose levels was causing me to feel lethargic.

for many Glucose Goddess community members, a glucose spike can also bring on poor mood or anxiety.

In the long term, the processes that spikes set into motion—oxidative stress, glycation, inflammation, and insulin excess—lead to chronic conditions, from type 2 diabetes to arthritis and depression.

SHORT-TERM EFFECTS

Constant hunger

Are you hungry all the time? You are not alone.

First, many of us feel hungry again shortly after we eat—and here again, it has to do with glucose. If you compare two meals that contain the *same number of calories*, the one that leads to a smaller glucose spike will keep you feeling full for longer. Calories aren't everything (more on this in part 3).

Second, constant hunger is a symptom of high insulin levels. When there is a lot of insulin in our body, built up over years of glucose spikes, our hormones get mixed up. *Leptin*, the hormone that tells us we are full and should stop eating, has its signal blocked, while *ghrelin*, the hormone that tells us we are hungry, takes over. Even though we have fat reserves, with lots of energy available, our body tells us we need more—so we eat.

As we eat, we experience more glucose spikes, and insulin rushes in to store excess glucose as fat, which then increases the action of ghrelin. The more weight we put on, the hungrier we get. It's an unfortunate, vicious, and unfair cycle.

The answer is not to try to eat less; it is to decrease our insulin levels by flattening our glucose curves—and this often actually means eating more food, as you'll see in part 3. There you'll hear the story of Marie, a community member who used to have to eat every 90 minutes and now doesn't even snack anymore.

Cravings

Our understanding of cravings changed thanks to an experiment that took place on the Yale University campus in 2011. Subjects were recruited and placed in an fMRI scanner, which measures brain activity. Then the subjects looked at photos of food on a screen—salad, burger, cookie, broccoli—and rated how much they wanted to eat them on a scale from 1 for "Not at all" to 9 for "Very much."

On a computer monitor, researchers watched which part of the subjects' brains activated as they looked at the photos.

The subjects had also given their consent to be hooked up to a machine that monitored their glucose levels.

What the researchers discovered was fascinating. When the subjects' glucose levels were stable, they didn't rate many of the foods highly. However, *when their glucose levels were decreasing*, two things happened: First, the craving center of their brain lit up when pictures of high-calorie foods were shown. Second, the participants rated those foods much higher on the "I want to eat it" scale than when their glucose levels were stable.

The finding? A decrease in glucose levels—even a small decrease of 20 mg/dL, which is less than the 30 mg/dL dip that occurs after we spike—makes us crave high-calorie foods.

The problem is, our glucose levels decrease all the time—specifically, they drop after every spike. And the higher the spike has been, the more intense the crash will be. That's good, because it means insulin is doing its job, stashing excess glucose in various storage units. But it also means that we're hit by a desire for a cookie or a burger—or both. Flattening our glucose curve leads to fewer cravings.

Chronic fatigue

Remember your grandfather and his terrible postretirement gig? When his cabin was stuffed with too much coal, he had to give up shoveling, and the train stopped. The same thing happens to our mitochondria: too much glucose makes them quit, energy production is compromised, and we are *tired*.

Experiments on stationary bikes show what happens when mitochondria don't work well: people born with mitochondrial defects can typically exercise only half as long as otherwise healthy people. If you have hurt mitochondria, picking your kid up is more challenging, carrying groceries is exhausting, and you won't be able to handle stress (such as a layoff or a breakup) as well as you used to. Difficult events, whether physical or mental, require mitochondria-generated energy to overcome.

When we eat something that tastes sweet, we may think that we are helping our body get energized, but it's just an impression caused by the dopamine rush in our brain that makes us feel high. With every spike, we are impairing the long-term ability of our mitochondria. Diets that cause glucose roller coasters lead to higher fatigue than those that flatten glucose curves.

Poor sleep

A common symptom of dysregulated glucose is waking up suddenly in the middle of the night with a pounding heart. Often, it's the result of a glucose crash in the middle of the night. Going to sleep with high glucose levels or right after a big glucose spike is also associated with insomnia in postmenopausal women and sleep apnea in a segment of the male population. If you want a good night's sleep, flatten your curves.

Colds and coronavirus complications

After a glucose spike, your immune system is temporarily faulty. If your glucose levels are chronically elevated, you can say goodbye to five-star immune responses against invaders—you will be more susceptible to infection, and this is particularly so, it turns out, in the case of the coronavirus. Good metabolic health (another way to describe how well your mitochondria are functioning) is one of the main factors that predict whether we'll survive a coronavirus infection; people with elevated glucose levels have been shown to be more easily infected, to more easily suffer complications, and to be more than twice as likely to die from the virus as people with normal glucose levels (41 percent versus 16 percent).

Gestational diabetes is harder to manage

In every woman, insulin levels increase during pregnancy. That's because insulin is responsible for encouraging growth—growth of the baby and growth of the mom's breast tissue so she can prepare to breastfeed.

Unfortunately, sometimes this extra insulin can lead to insulin resistance, meaning our body no longer responds to insulin as well as it once did. Our insulin levels rise, but that doesn't help stash excess glucose in the three "storage lockers" any better, and our glucose levels rise, too. This is what we call gestational diabetes. It's a scary experience for mothers, even more so because it gets worse as the baby's due date approaches.

But by flattening their glucose curves, mothers can reduce their likelihood of needing medication, reduce the birth weight of their baby (which is good because it makes birth easier and is healthier for the baby), and reduce the likelihood of a C-section, as well as limit their own weight gain during pregnancy. This is exactly what Amanda, whom you'll meet in part 3, was able to do.

Hot flashes and night sweats

As hormone levels drop dramatically in menopause, the changes can feel like an earthquake—everything is set off balance, and women experience symptoms from reduced libido to night sweats, insomnia, hot flashes, and more.

High or unstable glucose levels and high insulin levels make menopause feel worse. Research shows that hot flashes and night sweats, common symptoms of menopause, are more common in women who have high glucose and high insulin levels. But there's hope: a 2020 study from Columbia University found that flattening glucose curves is associated with fewer menopause symptoms, such as insomnia.

Migraine

Migraine is a debilitating condition, which comes in many forms. It's a young field of study, but data proves that women with insulin resistance are twice as likely to have regular migraine headaches than women who don't. When sufferers' insulin levels are lowered, things seem to get better: when treated with a medication that reduced the amount of insulin in the body, over half of a group of 32 people experienced a significant reduction in migraine frequency.

Memory and cognitive function issues

If you're about to take a test, balance a checkbook, or start an argument that you want to win, beware of what you eat just beforehand. It's easy to reach for something sweet when you want an energy boost, but this choice can affect your brain power. It turns out that big glucose spikes can impair memory and cognitive function.

This effect is worst first thing in the morning, after fasting throughout the night. I wish I had known this growing up, back when I ate a Nutella crepe for breakfast every day. If you have a 9 a.m. meeting in which you want to impress, eat a breakfast that will keep your glucose curve flat. See hack 4, "Flatten Your Breakfast Curve," in part 3.

Type 1 diabetes is harder to manage

Type 1 diabetes is an autoimmune condition in which people lose the ability to make insulin—the cells in their pancreas that control its production don't work.

Every time someone with type 1 diabetes experiences a glucose spike, their body cannot stash excess glucose in those three storage containers because there's no insulin to help. As a result, they need to inject themselves with insulin multiple times a day to compensate. But large spikes and dips are a daily, and stressful, challenge. By flattening their glucose curves, people with type 1 diabetes can lessen that challenge. Many things can get easier: they can exercise without fear of hypoglycemia (a state caused by low glucose levels), go to the bathroom less frequently (a side effect of glucose spikes), and even improve their mood.

All the hacks in part 3 apply to people with type 1 diabetes as well (and in hack 10 you'll read a story about Lucy, a type 1 diabetic, who successfully flattened her curves with the hacks). If you have type 1 diabetes, it's important to speak to your doctor before you embark on any dietary changes. Make sure your insulin dosage is adjusted if needed.

LONG-TERM EFFECTS

Acne and other skin conditions

Raise your hand if you wish you had known this in high school: starchy and sugary foods can set off a chain reaction that can show up as acne on your face and body and can even make your skin look visibly redder. This is because many skin conditions (including eczema and psoriasis) are driven by inflammation, which, as you learned, is a consequence of glucose spikes.

When we eat in a way that flattens our glucose curves, acne clears up, pimples get smaller, and inflammation is tamed. In a study in males aged 15 to 25, the diet that resulted in the flattest glucose curves led to a significant reduction in acne compared to a diet that caused glucose spikes. (Interestingly, they saw improvements even without reducing other foods known to contribute to acne, such as dairy products.)

Aging and arthritis

Depending on your diet, you may have spiked your glucose (and fructose) tens of thousands more times than your neighbor has by the time you reach 60. This will influence not just how old you *look externally* but how old you *are internally*. The more often we spike, the faster we age.

Glycation, free radicals, and the subsequent inflammation are responsible for the slow degradation of our cells—what we call *aging*. Free radicals also damage collagen, the protein found in many of our tissues, which causes sagging skin and wrinkles and can lead to inflammation in joints, rheumatoid arthritis, degradation of cartilage, and osteoarthritis: our bones get brittle, our joints are in pain, and we definitely can't go for a run in the park.

If there are too many free radicals and too much damage inside a cell, that cell can decide to undergo cell death to prevent further issues. But this isn't without consequences. When cells die, parts of us disappear: our bones waste away, our immune system weakens, our heart pumps less well, and neurodegenerative diseases such as Alzheimer's and Parkinson's can develop.

Flattening our glucose curves, along with exercising and reducing stress, is a potent way to prevent aging.

Alzheimer's and dementia

Of all organs, the brain uses the most energy. It's home to a *lot* of mitochondria. That means that when there is excess glucose in our body, our brain is vulnerable to the consequences. The neurons in our brain feel oxidative stress just as any other cells do: repeated glucose spikes, because they increase oxidative stress, lead to neuroinflammation and eventually cognitive dysfunction. On top of that, chronic inflammation is a key factor in almost all chronic degenerative diseases, including Alzheimer's.

Indeed, Alzheimer's and glucose levels are so closely connected that Alzheimer's is sometimes called "type 3 diabetes" or "diabetes of the brain." For instance, people with type 2 diabetes are four times more likely to develop Alzheimer's than nondiabetics. The signs are visible early, too: poorly controlled glucose in people with type 2 diabetes is associated with deficits in memory and learning.

Like the other symptoms mentioned here, it's possible that even cognitive decline is reversible: a growing number of studies show short-term and long-term improvements of memory and cognition when patients are put on a glucose-steadying diet. A therapeutic program out of UCLA found that after just three months of flattening their curves, people who had had to leave their jobs because of cognitive impairment were able to return to work and even perform better than before.

Cancer risk

Children born today have a one in two chance of developing cancer in their lifetime. And poor diet, together with smoking, is the main driver in 50 percent of cancers.

For starters, research documents that cancer may begin with DNA mutations produced by free radicals. Second, inflammation promotes cancer's proliferation. Finally, when there is more insulin present, cancer spreads even faster. Glucose is the key to many of these processes, and it shows in the data—people with fasting levels higher than 100 mg/dL, what is classified as prediabetes, have over double the likelihood of dying of cancer. Flattening glucose and insulin curves is thus an important step to helping prevent the development of cancer.

Depressive episodes

Your brain doesn't have sensory nerves, so when something is wrong, it can't alert you with pain as other organs do. Instead, you feel mental disturbances—such as poor mood.

When people eat a diet that leads to erratic glucose levels, they report worsening moods, more depressive symptoms, and more mood disturbances compared to those on a diet of similar composition but with steadier glucose levels. And the symptoms get worse as the spikes get more extreme, so any effort to flatten the curve, even moderately, could help you feel better.

Gut issues

It's in our gut that our food is processed, broken down into molecules absorbed into our blood or sent out to the garbage disposal. So it's no surprise that bowel distress—such as leaky gut, irritable bowel syndrome, and slowed intestinal transit—is linked to diet. The jury is still out on the link between glucose spikes and specific digestive issues, but it seems that high glucose levels could increase leaky gut syndrome. Indeed, inflammation—one of the processes set off by glucose spikes—can cause holes in the gut lining, so that toxins that aren't supposed to get through do (this is what leads to *leaky gut*). This in turn leads to food allergies and other autoimmune diseases, such as Crohn's disease and rheumatoid arthritis.

On another note, people who adopt a glucose-flattening diet can get rid of their heartburn or acid reflux very quickly—sometimes within one day.

What's more, we're discovering that gut health is linked to mental health—unhealthy microbiomes can contribute to mood disorders. The gut and the brain are connected by 500 million neurons (that's a lot, but the brain contains a whopping 100 billion). Information is sent back and forth between them all the time, which could be why what we eat, and whether or not we have glucose spikes, affects how we feel.

Heart disease

When we talk about heart disease, cholesterol is often the main topic of conversation. But that conversation is shifting; we've discovered that it isn't just a matter of "too much cholesterol." In fact, half the people who have a heart attack have *normal* levels of cholesterol. We now know that it's a specific type of cholesterol (LDL pattern B) as well as inflammation that drive heart disease. Scientists have found out why this is the case. And it's linked to glucose, fructose, and insulin.

First, glucose and fructose: The lining of our blood vessels is made of cells. Heart disease starts when *plaque* accumulates underneath that lining. These cells are particularly vulnerable to mitochondrial stress—and glucose and fructose spikes lead to oxidative stress. As a result, these cells suffer and lose their smooth shape. The lining of the vessels becomes bumpy, and fat particles get stuck more easily along the uneven surface.

Second, insulin: When our levels of insulin are too high, our liver starts producing LDL pattern B. This is a small, dense kind of cholesterol that creeps along the edges of the vessels, where it's likely to get caught. (LDL pattern A is large, buoyant, and harmless—we get it from eating dietary fat.)

Finally, if and when that cholesterol is oxidized—which happens the more glucose, fructose, and insulin are present—it lodges under the lining of our blood vessels and sticks there. Plaque builds up and obstructs the flow, and this is how heart disease starts.

Spikes drive these three processes. That's why science is finding that even if our fasting glucose is normal, each additional glucose *spike* increases our risk of dying of a heart attack. To help our heart, we should flatten our glucose, fructose, and insulin curves.

Nine out of ten doctors still measure *total* LDL cholesterol to diagnose heart disease and prescribe statins if it's too high. But what's important is LDL pattern B and inflammation. To add to the problem, statins lower LDL pattern A, but they don't lower the problematic pattern B. This is why statins don't decrease the risk of a first heart attack.

Here again, glucose and fructose, and the inflammation that high levels of these molecules cause in our bodies, are the key to understanding this disease. Doctors can better measure heart disease risk by looking at what's called the triglycerides-to-HDL ratio (which tells us about the presence of the small, dense LDL pattern B), and C-reactive protein (which tells us about inflammation levels).

Triglycerides become LDL pattern B in our bodies. So by measuring triglycerides, we can gauge the amount of the problematic LDL pattern B in our system. If you divide the level of triglycerides (in mg/dL) by HDL level (in mg/dL), you'll get a ratio that is surprisingly accurate in predicting LDL size. If the result is smaller than 2, that's ideal. If the result is above 2, it can be problematic. Then, because inflammation is a key driver of heart disease, measuring C-reactive protein, which increases as inflammation does, is better at predicting heart disease than cholesterol levels.

Infertility and polycystic ovarian syndrome (PCOS)

Scientists have recently discovered a remarkable connection between insulin and reproductive health. It turns out that insulin levels are an important piece of information used by the brain and your gonads, or sex organs, to decide whether your body is a safe environment in which to conceive. If your insulin is out of whack, your body isn't too keen on reproducing, because it suggests that you aren't healthy. Both women and men with high insulin levels are more likely to be infertile. The more glucose spikes in our diet, the higher our insulin levels and the higher our incidence of infertility.

When it comes to female infertility, polycystic ovarian syndrome (PCOS) is often to blame. One in eight women experience it, and when they do, their ovaries become burdened with cysts and no longer ovulate.

PCOS is a disease caused by too much insulin. The more insulin that is present, the more PCOS symptoms.

Why? Because insulin tells the ovaries to produce more testosterone (the male sex hormone). On top of that, with too much insulin, the natural conversion from male to female hormones that usually takes place is hampered—which leads to even more testosterone in the body. Because of the excess testosterone, women suffering from

PCOS display masculine traits: hair in places where they don't want hair (such as the chin), baldness, irregular or missed periods, or acne. Ovaries can also retain and accumulate eggs, stopping ovulation.

Many women with PCOS also have a hard time losing weight—because where there is too much insulin, there is an inability to burn fat.

Some women are more susceptible to PCOS than others (not every woman with high insulin levels has PCOS), but in all cases, keeping glucose levels under control can reduce and even alleviate symptoms. In part 3, you'll meet Ghadeer, who rid herself of PCOS symptoms, reversed her insulin resistance, and lost over 20 pounds using the hacks in this book. In a study performed at Duke University, women who went on a glucose level–flattening diet for six months cut their insulin levels by half and, as a consequence, their testosterone levels by 25 percent. Their body weight dropped and their body hair diminished as their hormones came into balance, and two of the 12 participants became pregnant in the course of the study.

For men, dysregulated glucose is also linked to infertility: elevated glucose levels are associated with reduced quality of semen (fewer viable candidates) and erectile dysfunction—so much so that recent studies point to the fact that erectile dysfunction in men under 40 years old could be due to an unknown metabolic and glucose dysregulation issue. If you are trying to get pregnant, flattening your glucose curves is a big help.

Insulin resistance and type 2 diabetes

Type 2 diabetes is a global epidemic, with half a billion people in the world suffering from the disease and the number rising every year. It's also the best-known health condition associated with elevated glucose levels. To better understand how spikes lead to type 2 diabetes and how to reverse the condition, let me tell you a story about my espresso habit.

When I was a student in London, I steadily increased my daily dose of coffee. I started with one espresso in the morning and after a few years somehow ended up at five a day just to stay awake. I had to keep upping my dose of caffeine to feel the same effect as before. In other words, I gradually became *resistant* to caffeine.

It's the same with insulin. When insulin levels have been high for a long time, our cells start becoming resistant to insulin. Insulin resistance is the root cause of type 2 diabetes: liver, muscle, and fat cells need larger and larger quantities of insulin to take up the same amount of glucose. Eventually, the system doesn't work anymore. Glucose is no longer stored away as glycogen, even though our pancreas produces growing quantities of insulin. The result is that the glucose levels in our body are increased for good. As our insulin resistance gets worse, we go from prediabetes (fasting glucose levels above 100 mg/dL) to type 2 diabetes (above 126 mg/dL). Slowly but surely, over many years, every glucose spike you experience will contribute to worsening your insulin resistance and raising the overall baseline glucose level in your body.

The common (but misguided) method of treating type 2 diabetes is to give the patient more insulin. This brings the glucose levels down temporarily by forcing the fat cells—that large storage container—to open (and make them put on weight). A vicious cycle is created, where higher and higher doses of insulin are administered and the patient's weight goes up and up, but the root problem of high insulin levels isn't addressed. Adding extra insulin helps type 2 diabetics in the short term, bringing their levels down after eating, but in the long term worsens the condition.

What's more, we now know that type 2 diabetes is an inflammatory disease—more inflammation, a process set off by glucose spikes, makes it worse.

It makes sense, therefore, that a diet that reduces our intake of glucose and therefore our production of insulin, would help reverse type 2 diabetes. A 2021 review of 23 clinical trials made it clear that the most effective way to reverse type 2 diabetes is to flatten our glucose curves. This is more effective than low-calorie or low-fat diets, for example (even though they can also work). In one study, type 2 diabetics who changed their diet and reduced their glucose spikes cut their insulin injections by *half* within one day. (If you are on medication, speak to your doctor before you try the hacks in this book—as you see, changes can be very rapid.)

In 2019, the American Diabetes Association (the ADA) started endorsing glucose-flattening diets in the light of compelling evidence that following these improves type 2 diabetes outcomes. Now we know that to reverse type 2 diabetes and insulin resistance, we need to flatten our glucose curves. In part 3, you'll learn how to do this while still eating what you love.

Nonalcoholic fatty liver disease

Liver disease used to be a problem only for those who drank a lot of liquor.

But in the twenty-first century, that changed. Robert Lustig, an endocrinologist, was confronted with a startling fact in his practice in San Francisco in the late 2000s: some of his patients were showing signs of liver disease, but they weren't heavy drinkers. In fact, many of them were under the age of 10.

He went on to discover that excess fructose could cause liver disease, just as alcohol does. To protect us from fructose, just as it does with alcohol, the liver turns fructose into fat, thereby removing it from the bloodstream. But when we repeatedly eat things high in fructose, our liver itself becomes *fatty*—which happens with alcohol, too.

The medical community named this new condition nonalcoholic fatty liver disease (NAFLD) or nonalcoholic steatohepatitis (NASH). It's extremely common: around the world, one out of every four adults has NAFLD. In people who are overweight, it's even more common: over 70 percent of them have it. Unfortunately, this condition can get worse over time, leading to liver failure or even cancer.

To reverse the condition, the liver needs a break so that it depletes its excess fat reserves. The solution to this is to lower our fructose levels and prevent further fructose spikes—which happens naturally when we flatten our glucose curves (because fructose and glucose go hand in hand in food).

Wrinkles and cataracts

Do you know why some 60-year-olds look as though they are 70, while others look as though they are 45? That's because we can influence the speed at which we age—and one of those ways is by flattening our glucose curves.

Glucose spikes, as I explained in the previous chapter, result in glycation—and glycation makes us age faster and look older.

For example, when glycation transforms a molecule of collagen, it makes it less flexible. Collagen is needed to repair wounds, as well as make healthy skin, nails, and hair. Broken collagen leads to sagging skin and wrinkles. The more glycation, the more sagging skin and wrinkles. Crazy but true.

Glycation happens everywhere in our body, including in our eyes; when it does, the molecules in our eyes experience damage and start to clump together. Over time, the accumulation of glycated proteins blocks the light and we develop cataracts.

~~~~~

Science, including the research I've shared here, helps you decode the messages from your body. Take a second and check in. How are you feeling? What parts hurt? Which systems feel sluggish? If you could wake up every day and feel amazing, wouldn't you want to?

Odds are, you are among the 88 percent of adults who have dysregulated glucose levels and experience, without knowing it, the many consequences of spikes I just described—from short-term side effects to long-term illnesses. From wrinkles and acne to cravings and hunger to migraine and depression and poor sleep to infertility and type 2 diabetes, these symptoms are messages from your body. And although these issues are very common, recent discoveries show us that they are also very much reversible.

In part 3, I show you how to start that process. You're about to discover food hacks that will help you flatten your curves, reconnect with your body, reverse your symptoms—while still eating what you love. I hope that soon you'll wake up one morning and feel amazing. Because that's exactly what happened to Bernadette, whom you're about to meet.

~~~~~

Note: If you take medication or insulin, it's important that you speak with your doctor before trying the hacks, because they can steady your glucose levels very quickly and your dosage might need to be adjusted.

PART 3

≈≈≈≈≈≈

How Can I Flatten
My Glucose Curves?

HACK 1 EAT FOODS IN THE RIGHT ORDER

"I lost five pounds in nine days," Bernadette told me on a sunny Tuesday morning, "and all I did was change the order in which I eat my food."

So often, we focus on *what* and *what not* to eat. But what about *how* to eat? It turns out that *how* we eat our food has a powerful effect on our glucose curves.

Two meals consisting of the same foods (and therefore the same nutrients and the same calories) can have vastly different impacts on our body depending on *how* their components are eaten. I was taken aback when I read the scientific papers that proved this, notably a seminal one out of Cornell University in 2015: if you eat the items of a meal containing starch, fiber, sugar, protein, and fat in a specific order, you reduce your overall glucose spike by 73 percent, as well as your insulin spike by 48 percent. This is true for anyone, with or without diabetes.

What is the right order? It's fiber first, protein and fat second, starches and sugars last. According to the researchers, the effect of this sequencing is comparable to the effects of diabetes medications that are prescribed to diabetics to lower their glucose spikes. A startling study from 2016 proved the finding even more definitively: two groups of type 2 diabetics were given a standardized diet for eight weeks and asked to either eat their food in the right order or eat it however they pleased. The group who ate their food in the right order saw a significant reduction in their HbA1c level, which means they started reversing their type 2 diabetes. The other group, eating the exact same food and number of calories but in no particular order, didn't see an improvement in their condition.

Talk about a groundbreaking discovery.

The explanation for this surprising effect has to do with how our digestive system works. In order to visualize it, think of your stomach as a sink and your small intestine as the pipe below it.

Anything you eat lands in your sink, then flows through to your pipe, where it is broken down and absorbed into your bloodstream. Every minute, on average, about three calories' worth of food trickles through from sink to pipe. (This process is called *gastric emptying*.)

If starches or sugars are the first thing to hit your stomach, they get to your small intestine very quickly. There, they are broken down into glucose molecules, which then make it through to the bloodstream very quickly. That creates a glucose spike. The more carbs you eat and the quicker you eat them, the more forcefully the load of glucose appears—the bigger the glucose spike.

Picture your stomach as a sink and your intestine as the pipe below it.

carbs
eaten first

When you eat carbs first, they flow into your intestine uninterrupted.

Say you have both pasta and vegetables on your plate (broccoli, anyone? I love broccoli) and you eat the pasta first, then the broccoli. The pasta, which is a starch, turns into glucose as it is quickly digested. The broccoli then "sits" on top of the pasta and waits its turn to go through the pipe.

On the other hand, consuming the *veggies first* and the *carbs second* significantly changes what happens.

Begin by munching on the broccoli. Broccoli is a vegetable, and vegetables contain plenty of fiber. As we've seen, fiber isn't broken down into glucose by our digestive system. Instead, it goes through from sink to pipe to . . . sewage, slowly and unchanged.

But that's not all.

Fiber has three superpowers: First, it reduces the action of alpha-amylase, the enzyme that breaks starch down into glucose molecules. Second, it slows down gastric emptying: when fiber is present, food trickles from sink to pipe more slowly. Finally, it creates a viscous

carbs eaten first

veggies eaten first

Eating veggies first and carbs second greatly slows down the speed at which glucose makes it to the bloodstream, thereby flattening the glucose spike associated with that meal.

mesh in the small intestine; this mesh makes it harder for glucose to make it through to the bloodstream. Through these mechanisms, fiber slows down the *breakdown* and *absorption* of any glucose that lands in the sink after it; the result is that fiber flattens our glucose curves.

Any starch or sugar that we eat *after fiber* will have a reduced effect on our body. We'll get the same pleasure from eating it but with fewer consequences.

That's carbs and vegetables. Now enter protein and fat. Protein is found in meat, fish, eggs, dairy, nuts, beans, and legumes. Foods that contain protein often contain fat, too, and fat is also found on its own in foods such as butter, oils, and avocados. (Incidentally, there are good and bad fats, and the bad fat that we should avoid is found in hydrogenated and refined cooking oils such as canola, corn, cottonseed, soybean, safflower, sunflower, grapeseed, and rice bran oil.) Foods containing fat also slow down gastric emptying, so eating them

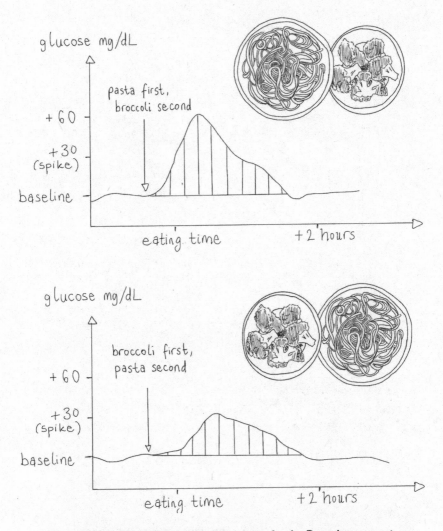

glucose mg/dL

pasta first,
broccoli second

+ 60

+ 30
(spike)

baseline

eating time   + 2 hours

glucose mg/dL

broccoli first,
pasta second

+ 60

+ 30
(spike)

baseline

eating time   + 2 hours

These two meals contain the exact same foods. But when we eat the vegetables first and the starch second, we flatten our glucose curve and experience fewer, and lesser, side effects of a glucose spike.

before rather than *after* carbs also helps flatten our glucose curves. The takeaway? Eating carbs after everything else is the best move.

To illustrate the effect of food order on glucose spikes, return to the Tetris analogy: blocks coming down slowly are easier to arrange than blocks coming down quickly. When we eat foods in the right

The right order to eat foods in: veggies first, protein and fat second, starch last.

order—veggies first, protein and fats second, carbs last—not only do we slow down the *speed* of the blocks, we even cut down on the *quantity* of blocks thanks to the mesh that fiber adds to our intestine. The slower the trickling of glucose into our bloodstream, the flatter our glucose curves and the better we feel. We can eat *exactly the same thing*—but by eating carbs last, we make a big difference in our physical and mental well-being.

What's more, when we eat foods in the right order, our pancreas produces less insulin. And as I explained in part 2, less insulin helps us return to fat-burning mode more quickly, the positive results of which are many—and include losing weight.

MEET BERNADETTE

Bernadette—who isn't diabetic—had been using this hack not because she wanted to lose weight (her girlfriends had warned her that postmenopausal pounds were impossible to shed) but simply because she wanted to feel better. Her attempt at weight loss had come to a halt a few years back. She was sick and tired of counting calories. She had tried intermittent fasting but it hadn't worked for her.

Now, at 57 years old, what bothered Bernadette most was her poor energy level. Every afternoon, like clockwork, she'd get so tired while going about her daily activities that she would glance at the floor at work, the bank, or the coffee shop, and think, *If only I could lie down there, I would have a fabulous nap.* To make it through the afternoon, she'd eat chocolate bars. But when it came to go to sleep at night, she suffered from insomnia, waking up around four every morning.

Bernadette first learned about glucose spikes on the Glucose Goddess Instagram account. She didn't know whether she was in fact experiencing spikes, but she decided to try this hack to see if it might help her.

When she found herself in her kitchen the next day at lunchtime, with the ingredients for her usual sandwich on her countertop, she recalled the "veggies first, protein and fat second, carbs last" hack and thought, *Hm. Instead of stacking everything and eating the sandwich*

Deconstruct a sandwich and eat the bread (starch) last to dampen the glucose spike it creates and get rid of the 3 p.m. sleepiness that comes when your glucose levels plummet.

as one, I could eat the salad and pickle first, then the tuna, then the toasted bread. She placed each on her plate and ate her newly baptized "deconstructed sandwich."

Bernadette is a creature of habit, and her go-to dinner is steak with veggies and pasta. So that day, she had the veggies and meat first and the pasta last. At no point did she change the quantity of food she was consuming—just the order in which she ate it.

The next day, to her great surprise, she woke up feeling rested for the first time in months. When she reached for her phone to check the time, she saw 7 a.m. — hours later than when she usually opened her eyes. I know this sounds crazy — Bernadette thought it was crazy, too. But she was thrilled. So she kept going, deconstructing her sandwiches and eating her pasta last in the evenings.

After three days, her longings for a midafternoon nap were gone. She was energized. She felt better than she had in years. When she went to the supermarket next, instead of stocking up on chocolate bars as she usually did, she didn't feel the need to buy any. "It was so freeing," she said.

TRY THIS: Next time you sit down for a meal, eat the veggies and proteins first and the carbs last. Note how you feel after eating compared to how you usually feel after a meal.

What was going on?

Before she changed the way she ate, Bernadette experienced the symptoms of a post-lunch glucose crash. She longed for a nap. Her brain sent a well-meaning, but incorrect, alert: *We're low on energy, we need to eat something.* She looked for a chocolate bar and promptly ate it. The chocolate bar caused her glucose levels to shoot right back up, after which they soon came falling down again. A wild roller-coaster ride.

When Bernadette changed the order of the food she ate, the spike it caused was smaller, so the drop was less pronounced. She felt less hungry and less tired in the afternoons. The roller-coaster ride came to a gentle stop.

There's a scientific explanation for this improvement in her hunger: the Cornell research team showed that if we eat our food in the

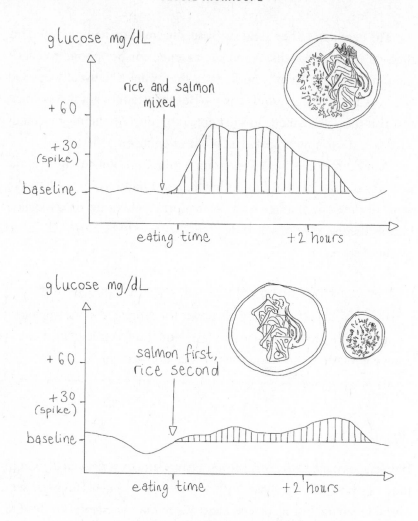

Even if there are no veggies on your plate, "deconstructing" your meals and eating carbs last helps your body. We significantly flatten the glucose curve and reduce the likelihood of weight gain, cravings, lethargy, and the harmful long-term side effects of elevated glucose levels.

wrong order (starches and sugars first), *ghrelin*, our hunger hormone, returns to premeal levels after just two hours. If we eat our food in the right order (starches and sugars last), ghrelin stays suppressed for much longer. (They didn't measure past three hours, but looking at the trends, I think it fair to say that it stays down for five to six hours.)

Research also shows that in postmenopausal women, a diet with fewer glucose spikes is associated with a lower incidence of insomnia. What's more, when we sleep better, we make better choices, and it's easier to find the motivation to do good for ourselves. Bernadette felt that way—she even started going for walks in the afternoon.

Nine days into what felt like the easiest lifestyle change she had ever tried, Bernadette's jeans started feeling looser. So she jumped on the scale. To her surprise, she was down five pounds. In just over a week, she had lost almost a third of the weight she had put on since menopause without even trying.

Remember, in the cockpit of our body, getting our glucose lever into the right position is the most powerful thing we can do. The consequences are often surprising, such as unintended weight loss. And as you see, it starts with something as easy as eating in the right order.

I thought fruit was supposed to be eaten alone, otherwise it rots in our stomach?

A question I am often asked when I talk about this hack involves fruit. I categorize fruits in the "sugars" category, because although they contain fiber, they are made up mostly of glucose, fructose, and sucrose—aka *sugars*. Therefore they should be eaten last. But people ask, "Doesn't eating fruit last cause it to rot in the stomach?" The short answer is no.

This false belief seems to date back to the Renaissance, around the time the printing press was invented. Some doctors at the time recommended that you should *never* finish a meal with raw fruit, because it would "float on top of the contents of the stomach and eventually putrefy, sending noxious vapours into the brain and disrupting the entire bodily system."

As it turns out, there is no evidence supporting this.

Rotting happens when bacteria lodges on food and starts digesting that food to fuel its own growth. The white and green specks you

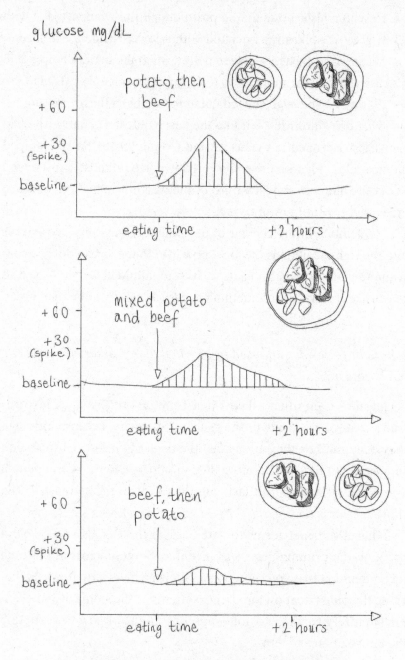

Eating the potato first led to the biggest spike, mixing it with the meat was better, but starting with the meat and saving the carbs for last was best for my glucose levels.

see on a strawberry you've left too long in the fridge are bacteria growing. First off, rotting takes days or weeks to happen. It can't happen in a few hours, which is about how long it takes for fruit to be digested. Second, our stomach is an acidic environment (pH 1–2), and any environment with a pH below 4 prevents bacterial overgrowth (and therefore rotting). Nothing can rot in the stomach, and in fact, the stomach, together with the esophagus, is the place where there are the *fewest* bacteria in our entire digestive tract.

Those Renaissance physicians didn't have it right. But there are many instances of cultures throughout history that have embraced the "right food order": in Roman times, a meal generally started with eggs and ended with fruit. During the Middle Ages in Europe, banquets usually ended with fruit to "close up digestion." Today, people in most countries end meals on a sweet note: dessert.

To be fair, maybe the doctors of the 1300s were not completely off the wall when they recommended that you eat fruit alone. A handful of people have shared with me that they have to eat fruit on its own; otherwise they experience discomfort, such as bloating or gas. It all comes back to listening to our body. Starches and sugars last are the right way to go, unless we personally feel that it doesn't agree with us.

How quickly can I eat the foods one after the other?

Many different timings were studied in clinical settings—0 minutes, 10 minutes, 20 minutes; they all seem to work. As long as you eat starch and sugars last, even if it's without stopping, you will flatten your glucose curve. During my meals, I just eat one food group right after the other (and so does Bernadette).

What if there aren't any starches or sugars in the meal?

Naturally, a meal with no starches or sugars will lead to only a very moderate glucose spike (some protein turns to glucose as well, but at a much lower rate than carbohydrates). However, it is still beneficial to start with veggies and have protein and fats second.

Do I have to do this all the time?

It's up to you to use the hacks in this book in a way that makes sense for you. In my own life, I eat foods in the right order when it's easy. If I'm eating a dish such as curry or paella, where veggies, proteins, fats, and carbs are mixed together and it's difficult to separate the ingredients, I don't stress about it. I sometimes have a few bites of veggies first, then eat the rest of the dish mixed.

The most important thing to remember is that it's best to eat starches and sugars *as late in the meal as possible.* And remember to celebrate the small changes: if you eat your veggies first, then mix starches with your protein and fat, that's still an improvement and is better than eating the veggies last.

LET'S RECAP

Whenever it's feasible and doesn't turn your meal into a complicated ordeal involving painstakingly separating the elements of the chef's special, it's best to eat anything that turns into glucose last. Start with the veggies and greens on your plate, then fat and protein, then starches and sugars. It's tempting to go straight for the carbs when you are hungry, but if you use this hack, your cravings will be curbed later on.

Based on the science, I love any meal that starts with a salad. Unfortunately, many dining experiences don't set us up for success: restaurants serve bread while you're waiting for food. Starting with starch is the absolute opposite of what you ought to do. It will lead to a glucose spike that you won't be able to tame, then a crash later on—which will intensify your cravings.

Now that I think of it, if I had to devise a way to get people to eat more at my restaurant, giving them the bread first is exactly what I would do.

HACK 2   ADD A GREEN STARTER TO ALL YOUR MEALS

I know what you're probably thinking as you read the title above: *This is the same as the previous hack, eat your veggies first.* No! This hack is on another level. I'm talking about *adding* a dish at the beginning of your meals. You will eat more than you usually do and flatten your glucose curves in the process (and in the next hack, we'll go over why adding these calories is good). The goal here is to return to how food used to be, before it was processed: wherever there were starches and sugars, there was also fiber. By adding a delicious green starter, we're bringing fiber back.

MEET JASS

A few years ago I finally got my mother the present she had always wanted: a card that read "OMG—My mom was right about everything!"

To be fair, she wasn't right about starting the day with Special K and orange juice at breakfast. But she *was* right about some other things, such as the importance of organizing my mail, not buying clothes that needed to be dry-cleaned because I'd never get around to dropping them off, and scrubbing the inside of the fridge once a month. But when I first left home and went to college, I didn't follow any of that advice. I sure as heck didn't clean the inside of any kitchen appliances.

As we age, we often realize the wisdom of our parents' advice. As I've studied the science behind glucose spikes, I've seen multiple studies showing that some recommendations for flattening our glucose curves are ones that were encouraged by the previous generation.

That's what Jass discovered, too.

Jass (short for Jassmin) grew up in the countryside of Sweden with a Lebanese mother and a Swedish father. Her parents were busy: they had full-time jobs and five children. But no matter how busy they were, the family sat down to eat together every night. The first course of each dinner was always a large salad.

When Jass moved out and got her first job as a teacher in Gothenburg, just like me, she didn't think to follow her family's example. Her days were paced by the back-and-forths between her apartment and the middle school. She was swamped by coursework and, in between deadlines, tried to maintain her social life—in short, she didn't have time to think about food. Her usual tactic was to swing by the grocery store on her way home from work, pick up a box of pasta, and eat that for dinner. She'd pack the leftovers for lunch the next day.

Before she knew it, her eating habits had completely changed. Once someone who just enjoyed chocolate for dessert, she had now developed a sweet tooth. She counted the seconds until break when she could go to the coffee shop and buy a slice of cake. She needed a regular supply of treats to get through the day. The new job was taxing, she worked a lot and was quite tired, and eating something sweet every few hours kept her motivated.

As the months went on, her sweet tooth grew even more pronounced. She was either eating sugar or thinking about eating sugar. Her cravings were out of control. And in fact, her cravings were controlling her. Her willpower was nowhere to be found. She started to gain weight. Acne appeared on her forehead. Her periods became irregular. She felt bad—about the cravings and all the changes taking place in her brain and her body.

One afternoon, before Jass's usual snack time, she asked her class to open their biology books to chapter 10, "Metabolism." She spoke about how our body gets energy from food and in particular what happens when we eat carbohydrates. Jass was teaching a lesson on glucose.

As she went through the material, she couldn't help but think that maybe there was something that could help her here. In the same week, serendipitously, a colleague showed her the Glucose Goddess Instagram account. Things started clicking. She wondered: Is glucose the problem? Am I experiencing glucose spikes without knowing it? Is this why I can't stop eating chocolate and why I feel so tired all the time?

She soon noticed two things: (1) when she was hungry, she always went for carbs first and (2) her meals weren't balanced: lunch and dinner were mostly starches. She realized she was getting messages from her body: something was off. Yes, she was definitely on a glucose roller coaster.

In order to flatten our glucose curves, eating fiber, protein, and fat before starchy foods is key. With this empowering realization, Jass decided to reinstate a tradition from back home: a first course every night of a large salad. She had grown up eating fattoush, a traditional Lebanese salad. So off she went to make it herself: she combined chopped bell peppers, cucumbers, tomatoes, and radishes with lettuce, a handful of parsley, spring onions, and seasoned it with olive oil, salt, and a lot of lemon juice.

THE MORE FIBER, THE BETTER

The amount of fiber we eat these days is much lower than what we should be eating. Only 5 percent of Americans meet the recommended daily amount: 25 grams per day. The US government calls it a "nutrient of public health concern." This disappearance is due mostly to food processing, as I explained in part 1.

Fiber is in the structural lining of plants—it's abundant in leaves and bark. So unless you're a wood-eating termite (in which case, I'm

Beans, leafy greens, and veggies are great sources of fiber.
We need to be eating more of it, as it helps curb glucose spikes.

impressed that you can read!), you get most of your fiber from beans, vegetables, and fruit.

This plant-made substance is incredibly important to us: it fuels the good bacteria in our gut, strengthens our microbiome, lowers our cholesterol levels, and makes sure everything runs smoothly. One of the reasons a diet high in fruit and vegetables is healthy is because of the fiber it provides.

As mentioned in the last hack, fiber is also good for our glucose levels for several reasons, notably because it creates a viscous mesh in our intestine. The mesh slows down and reduces the absorption of molecules from food across the intestinal lining. What does this mean for our glucose curves? First, that we absorb fewer calories (we'll talk about calories in the next hack). Second, with fiber in our system, any absorption of glucose or fructose molecules is lessened.

This has been shown many times in scientific settings. For instance, in a 2015 study, scientists in New Zealand fed participants two types of bread: regular bread and enriched bread with 10 grams of fiber per serving. They found that the additional fiber reduced the glucose spike of the bread by over 35 percent. Talking about bread, here's what you're looking for if you want to enjoy some while

Want bread with
beneficial fiber
in it? Go for the
German ones.

flattening your curves: skip the loaves that claim to contain "whole grain," which often don't have much more fiber than their traditional "white" counterparts. Buy bread that is dark and dense, made from rye with a sourdough starter. It's traditionally German and usually called *seed bread* or *pumpernickel*. Those contain the most fiber.

However, even this dark bread is not the best way to add fiber to our diet, as bread contains starch and always leads to a glucose spike. You know what's a better way to get fiber? Green veggies. These contain mostly fiber and very little starch.

We know that consuming more fiber is beneficial and that eating it *before* all the other foods is even more so (see previous hack). That's why adding a green starter to each of our meals has a powerful effect on our glucose curves.

How big should this green starter be? As big as you like. I've found that the sweet spot is a one-to-one ratio to the carbs you'll eat after. My favorite: two cups of spinach, five jarred artichoke hearts, vinegar, and olive oil. My little brother's go-to: one big raw carrot, sliced, with hummus (not technically *green* but still vegetable-based, which is what we're looking for). You'll find more ideas later in this hack.

Around the world, tradition mirrors science: in Iran and the countries of Central Asia, meals start with fresh herbs eaten by the bunch. Around the Mediterranean, meals open with vegetables—marinated eggplant and artichokes for antipasti in Italy, sliced radishes, spring beans, and more as crudités in France, or the combination of finely

We can add any type of vegetables as our starter.
This includes vegetables that aren't green, such as carrots.
You can throw in some beans, too, such as hummus or
lentils, because they are full of fiber as well.

chopped parsley with ripe tomatoes and cucumbers that makes up tabbouleh from Turkey to Lebanon and Israel. Adding a green starter flattens our glucose curve. With a flatter curve, we stay full longer and avoid the glucose dip that leads to cravings a few hours later.

So back to Jass.

Jass hadn't realized that when she ate pasta on its own, she got onto a glucose roller coaster. By adding a salad at the beginning of every meal, she flattened her glucose curve. Her uncontrollable cravings dampened, and her willpower came back.

Jass added fattoush as a starter to her dinner each night. She still ate her usual bowl of pasta after, but now something different was happening in her body: She went from a forceful delivery of glucose to a gentle one. The spike was less pronounced, and the crash that followed was smaller.

Pretty quickly, Jass began to feel better. First, and most noticeable to her, she was able to go longer without eating. After lunch, she felt full until 5 p.m., instead of feeling ravenous at 3 p.m. She was more alert. She had more patience with her students. She found herself skipping through the hallways and smiling at her colleagues. The flatter curve had steadied both her hunger and her mood.

About 10 days in, Jass lost her taste for treats. To her great surprise, on her coffee break, she could walk by the local bakery and think, *Oh, a tasty-looking cake*, without feeling the urge to eat it. There was the *habit* of eating sweets but no torturous impulse to act on it. She didn't need to spend energy trying to suppress her cravings anymore—because her cravings were gone. She regained her willpower—in fact, it now felt like a superpower.

When we flatten our glucose curves, the side effects are usually pleasant and unexpected. As in the case of Bernadette, Jass lost weight without trying. So far she's lost 20 pounds, going from 183 pounds to 163. "I just cared about keeping my body in a happy steady glucose zone. Everything else fell into place." She told me that her period is back to normal, her acne has cleared up, she sleeps better, and she feels better, too.

TRY THIS: Think of your favorite veggie or salad. Prepare it with care, and eat it before every lunch and dinner for a week. Notice your cravings and whether they change.

How much time do I need to wait between the starter and the main dish?

You don't need to wait at all; you can eat them in sequence. If you do wait, try not to wait more than a couple of hours between your green starter and the rest of your meal. That's because two hours is around the time it takes for fiber to go through our stomach and the top part of our small intestine. For example, if you have a salad at noon and rice at 1 p.m., the fiber from the salad will still help flatten the rice's spike. But if you have a salad at noon and rice at 3 p.m., the salad won't help flatten the spike from the rice anymore.

How many veggies do I need to eat?

First off, any amount is better than none, and the more, the better. Studies haven't been done on the ideal ratio. But I try to eat the same quantity of veggies as the starches that follow.

If I don't have time to make a salad, I grab two jarred hearts of palm or a couple pieces of roasted cauliflower that I keep in the fridge. Though that's not a one-to-one ratio, it's enough to start seeing a small benefit, and it's better than having no veggies before a meal at all.

What qualifies as a green starter?

Any vegetable qualifies, from roasted asparagus to coleslaw to grilled zucchini and grated carrots. We're talking artichokes, arugula, broccoli, brussels sprouts, eggplant, lettuce, pea shoots, and tomatoes, and also pulses, beans, and viscous foods such as natto (a Japanese food made from soybeans)—the more, the better.

Incidentally, you can eat them either raw or cooked. But skip juiced or mashed preparations, because the fiber in them is either missing (in the case of a juice) or blitzed to oblivion (in the case of a mash). Soup is another story. Do you remember my answer to my mother when she calls me from the grocery store to ask if a food is "good" or "bad"? The answer is relative—and soup is a perfect example of this. Soup is a great dish—it contains plenty of nutrients and vitamins, it's filling, and it's one of the healthiest starters you can order at a restaurant. But it's not healthier than eating a whole vegetable. Beware of store-bought soups, too: they are often mostly potatoes, which breaks down into starch, and lots of added sugar.

What's the easiest thing to start with?

Buy a bag of spinach at the supermarket, toss 3 cups of it in a bowl with 2 tablespoons of olive oil, 1 tablespoon of vinegar (any kind you like), and salt and pepper, and top with a handful of crumbled feta cheese and toasted nuts. (It's okay, and good, to mix some protein and fats into your green starter.) You can also add pesto, grated parmesan cheese, and some toasted seeds, as you prefer. It should be something quick that you find tasty. This isn't cooking; it's assembling.

Beware of premade dressings, as they're often packed with sugar and loaded with vegetable oil—it's better to make a simple one from scratch with the ratio of oil and vinegar I describe above. I make a batch of dressing every Sunday and keep it in the fridge to use all week.

Here are some even quicker things to eat:

- A couple of pieces of leftover roasted veggies (top tip: I often roast a batch of broccoli or cauliflower and keep it in the fridge)
- A few mouthfuls of pickled vegetables
- A sliced cucumber with guacamole
- A sliced tomato with one or two slices of mozzarella cheese
- Baby carrots with hummus
- Four marinated artichokes from a jar or any other jarred veggies
- Two canned hearts of palm
- Two spears of jarred white asparagus

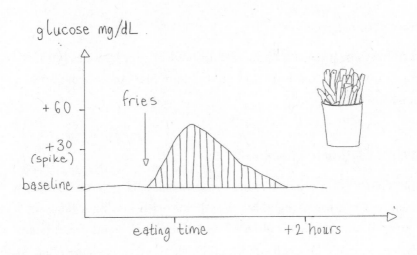

glucose mg/dL

+ 60

+ 30
(spike)

baseline

fries

eating time   + 2 hours

glucose mg/dL

+ 60

+ 30
(spike)

baseline

side salad,
then fries

eating time   + 2 hours

**When you are out at a restaurant and aren't ordering starters,
the main course side salad with olive oil and vinegar is your best ally.
Order it, then eat it first. The fiber and fat will make
any further starch arrival much smoother for your body.**

What about calories?

Great question. More on that in the next hack. Stay tuned.

How about supplements?

It's always best to eat whole food instead of supplements, but if it's easier on some occasions, a fiber supplement at the beginning of a meal can help.

What do I do at a restaurant?

If my party is ordering starters, I order a salad. If we aren't ordering starters, I ask for a vegetable-based side with my main (such as a simple green salad with olive oil and vinegar, steamed green beans, sauteed spinach, or even simmered black, navy, or garbanzo beans), and I eat it before the rest of my dish. I wait until after eating my veggies to eat my main or touch the bread.

Doesn't adding fat (from the salad dressing) to carbs lead to weight gain?

It doesn't—that's a myth that's been debunked. More on that in hack 10, "Put some clothes on your carbs."

MEET GUSTAVO AND HIS WINGMAN, BROCCOLI

People around the world get creative when they use these hacks in their daily lives. Depending on the country and what is available, their interpretations always impress me. I'd like to mention one example of how this hack helped Gustavo, because I find it particularly useful.

Gustavo is a salesman in Mexico. At 50, he has already lost two people close to him to the same disease: his father passed away from type 2 diabetes; then his colleague—years younger—also died of diabetes complications. That was a wake-up call. Gustavo didn't want his life to end because of poor health; he wanted to be an active member of his community for many years to come.

Gustavo hadn't (yet) been diagnosed with diabetes, but he knew he was seriously overweight, and, when he learned that people can experience spikes for years before developing the condition, he was pretty sure he was on his way there, just like his dad. That said, he also learned that diabetes isn't just about genes: even if our parents get diabetes, this does not mean that we automatically get it, too. Our DNA can increase our likelihood of getting it, but our lifestyle is still the main reason we do—or don't.

After discovering the Glucose Goddess Instagram account and learning about glucose and diabetes, Gustavo was ready for change, but the main barrier to it was his social life: when he went out for dinner, he would follow along with his party and eat a lot of starches and sugars. He wanted to change his habits, but the judgment of his friends was difficult to deal with. "Why are you ordering a salad?" they asked. "Are you on a *diet*?"

So he devised a trick: before going out for dinner, at home, he made himself a big plate of grilled broccoli and ate it with salt and hot sauce.

With broccoli in his belly, he was ready for his meal out. When he got to a restaurant, he wasn't starving, so he could easily forgo the bread on the table. And anyway, the effect of whatever starch and sugar he now ate would be curbed by the broccoli. That meant less of a glucose spike and less insulin release, along with less inflammation, less damage to his cells, and less inching toward type 2 diabetes.

Eighteen months into his glucose journey, Gustavo has lost 88 pounds. You'll learn about the other hacks he implemented in later chapters. When we spoke on the phone, he happily told me that he feels younger than ever. He can now run five miles without pain, something he had never been able to do but had always dreamed of. Beyond his physical improvements, Gustavo also shared that he

If you aren't sure you're going to be able to have a green starter at a restaurant, you can eat one before going out. Gustavo eats a large head of broccoli at home before meeting his friends at the steak house.

felt more confident and better informed than ever: he explained that finally, he understands that *calories aren't everything.*

HACK 3 STOP COUNTING CALORIES

If you follow the hack from the previous chapter, you will start adding calories to your meal in the form of a green starter. If you're hoping to shed pounds, you may wonder: Is that really a good idea? Won't adding calories make me gain weight? The short answer is no. The long answer involves understanding more about the *types* of calories we're eating—and lighting things on fire.

To measure how many calories are in, say, a doughnut, here's what to do: dehydrate the doughnut, and place it in a cubicle submerged in a water bath. Then light the doughnut on fire (yes, really) and measure by how many degrees the water around it warms up. Multiply the temperature change by the amount of water in the

thermometer
ignition wires
water
oxygen atmosphere
doughnut in container

To measure the calories in a doughnut, we measure how much it warms water up when burned.

container, the energy capacity of water (which is 1 calorie per gram per degree), and you'll get the number of calories in the doughnut.

So when we say "This doughnut and this Greek yogurt have the same number of calories," we're really saying "This doughnut and this Greek yogurt warm up water by the same number of degrees when we burn them."

It's through this burning technique—called a *calorimeter* and first invented in 1780—that scientists can measure the calories in anything. The coal that your grandfather shovels onto the fire stands proudly at 3.5 *million* calories per pound (because it burns very slowly and releases a lot of heat). A 500-page book, on the other hand, isn't the best choice if you're trying to heat water: it contains only *half a calorie* (because a book turns to ashes very quickly and in the process doesn't produce much heat).

In any case, calories measure heat generated, nothing else.

Judging a food based on its calorie count is like judging a book by its page count. The fact that a book is 500 pages long can certainly give you some information about how long it will take to read (about 17 hours), but it's unfortunately reductive. If you walk into a bookstore and tell an employee you want to buy "a 500-page book," they will look at you a little strangely and then ask for clarification. One 500-page book is not the same as another 500-page book, and likewise one calorie isn't the same as another.

One hundred calories of fructose, 100 calories of glucose, 100 calories of protein, and 100 calories of fat may release the same amount of heat when they burn, but they have vastly different effects on your body. Why? Because they are different *molecules*.

Here's this fact in action: in 2015, a research team out of UC San Francisco proved that we can keep eating the exact same number of calories, but if we change the *molecules* we eat, we can heal our body of disease. They demonstrated, for example, that calories from fructose are worse than calories from glucose (it's because fructose, as you know from part 2, inflames our bodies, ages our cells, and turns to fat more than glucose does).

This study involved obese teenagers. They were asked to replace the calories in their diet that came from fructose with calories from glucose (they replaced fructose-containing foods such as doughnuts with foods containing glucose but no fructose such as bagels). The number of calories they consumed was kept constant. What happened? Their health improved: their blood pressure improved, and their triglycerides-to-HDL ratio (a key marker of heart disease, as we learned in part 2) improved. They started reversing the progression of their fatty liver and their type 2 diabetes. And this profound change in their health happened in *just nine days*.

The results were conclusive: 100 calories of fructose are worse for us than 100 calories of glucose. This is why it's always better to eat something starchy than something sweet—more on that in hack 9, "If you have to snack, go savory." If the study had cut fructose and replaced it with protein, fat, and fiber (if the participants had replaced the doughnuts with Greek yogurt and grilled broccoli, for example), you can imagine that the effects would have been even more positive.

So if you've ever heard that to get healthy you just need to cut calories, now you know that's not true. You can do much to heal your body by changing the molecules you eat but keeping the calories the same.

How about weight loss—is it just a matter of consuming fewer calories? We used to think so, but that myth has been debunked, too. And there is a clue in the study I mentioned above: several of the teenagers started losing weight even though they were eating the same number of calories as before. Impossible? No—but it definitely goes against what we have been told for years.

In fact, recent science shows that people who focus on flattening their glucose curves can eat *more* calories and lose *more* fat *more*

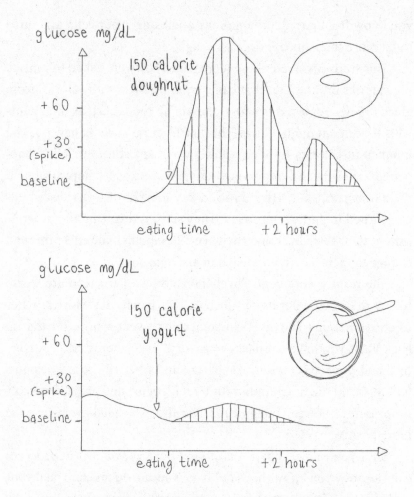

Same calories, different effects. The calories from the doughnut (containing fructose) were preferentially converted to fat, inflamed my body, and aged my cells. The calories from the yogurt (no fructose) did so much less.

easily than people who eat fewer calories but do not flatten their glucose curves. Let's repeat that: people on a glucose-flattening diet can lose more weight *while eating more calories* than people who eat fewer calories but spike their glucose levels.

For instance, a 2017 study from the University of Michigan showed that when overweight subjects focused on flattening their glucose curves (even if they ate *more* calories than the other group did), they lost more weight (17 pounds versus 4 pounds) than the subjects who ate fewer calories and took no care with their blood sugar levels.

It has to do with insulin: when we decrease our glucose levels, our insulin levels come down, too. A 2021 review analyzing 60 weight loss studies proved that insulin reduction is primordial and always precedes weight loss.

In fact, it seems that we can completely ignore calories and still lose weight if we just focus on flattening our glucose curves. Keep in mind that this needs to be done with a little bit of good judgment (if you eat 10,000 calories of butter a day, your glucose curves will be flat, but you'll gain weight). The feedback on this from Glucose Goddess community members has been pretty much universal: if they take care not to spike their glucose levels, they can eat until they feel full, without counting calories, and still lose weight.

That was exactly what Marie did, and it changed her life.

MEET MARIE: SHE CAN'T STOP SNACKING

Twenty-eight-year-old Marie lives in Pittsburgh and works in operations at a tech company. For almost a decade, every time she left the house, she tucked a purse full of snacks under her arm. That was non-negotiable: if she didn't eat every 90 minutes, she would start feeling shaky and spacy and need to sit down. Her diary was organized around that requirement—if an event lasted longer than an hour and a half and she knew she wouldn't be able to eat during it, she would not attend. (She made an exception for her niece's baptism—but ate a cereal bar right before she entered the church and ran to her car at the end to open a bag of chips.)

Many of us know someone (or indeed, *are* someone) who doesn't feel well if they don't eat at very specific intervals. People who experience this will sometimes say "I have low blood sugar." This is not necessarily incorrect—but what they might not know is that this isn't a condition they were born with. More often than not, their low blood sugar is caused by the insulin released after a previous snack. What would be more accurate would be to say "My glucose levels are crashing."

Usually, when insulin ushers glucose to the "storage lockers" after a spike, the curve is smooth and bell-shaped and glucose is brought back down steadily to its fasting level.

Sometimes, however, our pancreas releases too much insulin. As a result, too much glucose is stashed away. Instead of our glucose coming back down to fasting levels, it actually crashes and goes below normal for a little bit.

This is called *reactive hypoglycemia.* When our glucose level dips and before our body brings it back up by releasing extra glucose into the blood, we can feel side effects: hunger, cravings, shakiness, light-headedness, or tingling in our hands and feet. Which was how Marie felt many times throughout the day.

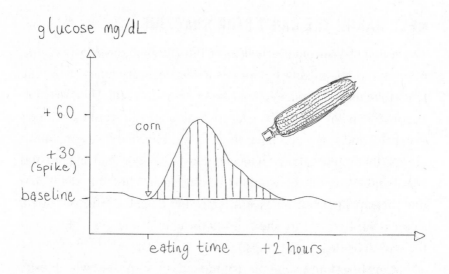

This is an example of insulin bringing glucose levels back down to normal after eating. After the spike, glucose went back down to its baseline level.

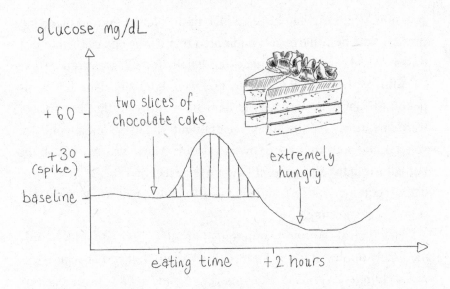

glucose mg/dL

+ 60 —

+30 —
(spike)

baseline —

two slices of
chocolate cake

extremely
hungry

eating time   +2 hours

**This is an example of reactive hypoglycemia and the hunger produced by it.
After the spike, glucose levels crashed down way below baseline level.**

Reactive hypoglycemia is a common condition, especially in people with other glucose-related issues such as PCOS. How little or how much you experience it varies widely. In people with diabetes, the swings of reactive hypoglycemia tend to be more pronounced—and their glucose level can get so low that it causes a coma. In nondiabetics, just a small dip can lead to extreme hunger, even if a meal was only two hours ago. And the greater the dip, the more hungry we become before the next meal.

A doctor's test confirmed that Marie did indeed have reactive hypoglycemia. (The test involves drinking a shake with a lot of glucose in it and getting your blood values tested for three hours afterward to detect the drop below baseline.)

This diagnosis was added to the long list of health conditions that Marie had received since her teenage years: hypothyroidism, psoriatic arthritis, estrogen dominance, candida infections, rashes, psoriasis, leaky gut, chronic fatigue, insomnia, nighttime anxiety. On one occasion, when she had gone to pick up her latest thyroid medicine prescription, her pharmacist had noted that it was one of the highest doses he had ever compounded—especially for a 28-year-old.

Still, Marie tried her best to feel well. And since she felt compelled to snack throughout the day, she made sure that her snacks were "healthy." At the time, she thought "healthy" meant mostly vegetarian foods that were low in calories. Marie was careful about her calorie intake in general (she never exceeded the 2,000-calorie daily recommendation), and she also forced herself to walk 10,000 steps every morning.

Her typical day went something like this: Fruit and granola immediately upon waking at 5 a.m. (she woke up that early because she was so hungry). Low-fat fruit yogurt at 6 a.m. A 100-calorie pack of cereal at 8 a.m. A Pop-Tart at 9:30 a.m. A vegetarian wrap at 11 a.m. A vegetarian sandwich for lunch with coconut water and a 100-calorie

This graph represents the glucose curve of someone with a diagnosis like Marie's—lots of spikes and dips below normal levels, called *reactive hypoglycemia.*

pack of pretzels, then a 100-calorie pack of cookies 90 minutes later. At 4 p.m. every day she ate a full pound of grapes—that's about 180 grapes. Crackers an hour before dinner, lots of rice and some beans for dinner, then a piece of chocolate before bed.

She was eating the "right" number of calories, but she was hungry all the time. She was chronically fatigued and couldn't muster the energy to do anything past noon every day. She was so tired that she drank *10 cups of coffee a day*.

When people get a reactive hypoglycemia diagnosis, they often hear that they should snack every few hours to make sure their glucose doesn't drop too low. But this just makes the problem worse: they eat something sweet or starchy, which shoots their glucose back up, releases insulin, and makes their levels come crashing down again. Then the cycle repeats. They're on a never-ending glucose roller coaster.

A more effective way to combat reactive hypoglycemia (which is a reversible condition, by the way) actually addresses the root problem: too much insulin. The solution is—you guessed it—to flatten the patient's glucose curve. With smaller spikes, that patient releases less insulin and experiences smaller dips. The body learns to not expect starchy and sweet snacks every few hours and, with less insulin present, starts burning fat reserves for fuel. It's important to make this change away from starchy and sweet snacks gradually, because it can take a few days or even weeks for the body to adapt.

That was what Marie desperately needed to do to feel better. Thankfully, while researching the meaning of *glycemia* and going down an internet rabbit hole, she found her way to my Instagram account.

She learned that when we flatten our glucose curves (and therefore our insulin curves), our reactive hypoglycemia goes away, because reactive hypoglycemia is a symptom of a glucose-spiking diet.

So Marie made some changes. Her plan was to eat as much as she felt was necessary as long as she kept her glucose curves flat.

She ate her carbs last, added salads to her meals, and introduced more protein, fat, and fiber into her diet. She switched from mostly processed foods, made of sugars and starches and devoid of fiber, to mostly whole foods, with lots of fiber. She wasn't counting calories anymore, but she definitely ate more than the 2,000 calories she used to.

Now, for breakfast, she has oatmeal with ground flax seeds, hemp seeds, nuts, pea protein powder, and a sausage on the side. At lunchtime, two hard-boiled eggs, carrot sticks, celery, peanut butter or avocado, a protein smoothie (with collagen powder, 1 tablespoon of chia seeds, half a tablespoon of coconut oil, and a whole bunch of greens), and half a banana last. For a snack in the afternoon, Greek yogurt, berries, and half a protein bar. Finally, at dinner, fish or chicken, kale sautéed with avocado oil, and roasted sweet potatoes.

Marie shared the good news on the phone with me: "I've been able to go *four hours* without a meal! I can even exercise fasted. That has given me my life back!"

That starving sensation every few hours quickly became a thing of the past. So did her reactive hypoglycemia. Other things changed, too. Marie's energy levels increased within a week or two, to the point where she went from 10 cups of coffee a day to one. Her skin breakouts cleared up; her rashes and psoriasis, too. Her headaches disappeared. So did her insomnia, panic attacks, and psoriatic arthritis. Her estrogen levels returned to normal levels. She lost about five pounds.

Her thyroid functioning improved as well. Every couple of months, her doctor administered tests and adjusted her meds to lower and lower dosages. Her pharmacist doesn't remark on her prescription anymore.

And almost best of all? She no longer carries snacks in her purse.

This is what Marie's daily glucose levels look like now: small variations within the healthy range, with no more reactive hypoglycemia. She eats more calories than before, and she feels so much better.

She doesn't need to. That may seem like a small thing, but to Marie, it changed everything.

So remember this: health and weight loss have more to do with what molecules you ingest than the number of calories in what you eat.

What does this mean for us?

It means we can, without fear, add calories to a meal if the calories help curb the glucose spike of that meal: i.e., if the molecules are fiber, fat, or protein. When we add a dressed salad to a meal, the calories we add are helpful to us, because they help keep our glucose and insulin levels low and even help us absorb fewer calories from what we eat after the salad (due to the mesh that fiber creates). On balance, we stay full longer, can burn more fat, and put on less weight.

Flip the logic around: if we add more glucose or fructose to a

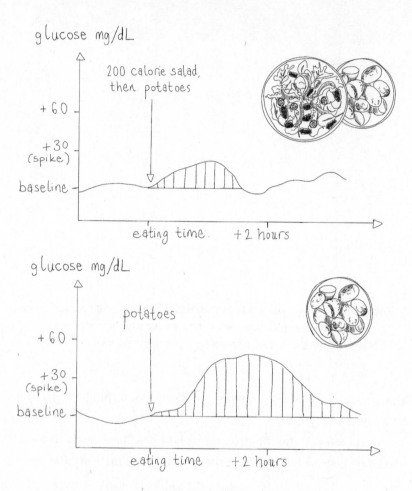

When we add a 200-calorie salad (fiber and fat) to a meal, we are adding calories to it, but those calories help curb the glucose and insulin spikes. Those are good calories to add.

meal, this *increases* the spikes, which leads to more weight gain, more inflammation, and less satiety.

The fact that all calories are not equal is something that the processed food industry does its best to obfuscate. It hides behind calorie counts because they divert our attention away from scrutinizing what's actually *in the box*—such as lots of fructose, which, unlike glucose, cannot be burned by our muscles for fuel and is almost all

When we add a 200-calorie soda (glucose and fructose) to a meal, those calories amplify the spikes: in fact, they increase the concentrations of the big three—glucose, fructose, and insulin. Those aren't good calories to add.

converted postdigestion into fat. Look at the "shout lines" on snack packets when you next go to the store, and you will see what I mean. Food manufacturers keep asserting that all calories are the same, because the truth is a threat to their interests. It's an easy trick.

This is exactly how Special K became a commercial success, perceived by consumers as the quintessential weight loss cereal: the box proudly touted "Just 114 calories!" We didn't think twice about it, and we didn't know that, even though it was relatively low in calories, Special K contained twice the amount of sugar as other cereals such as corn flakes. We didn't know that those 114 calories of sugar and starch would lead to a glucose spike and an insulin spike—and certainly more fat gain than 114 calories from, say, eggs and toast. We didn't know that those 114 calories of Special K for breakfast would start us on a glucose roller coaster—and lead to cravings all day long. But now, thanks to continuous glucose monitors and curious scientists—which I'll tell you about next—we have proof that cereal for breakfast is definitely, unequivocally not a good way to start the day.

HACK 4 FLATTEN YOUR BREAKFAST CURVE

The campus of Stanford University in California is home to a team of scientists who specialize in the study of continuous glucose monitoring. In 2018, they did something that all great scientists do: they challenged assumptions. Specifically, they set out to test the commonly accepted belief that, unless you are diabetic, your glucose levels should be of no concern. Second, and perhaps more controversially, they wanted to test a practice that has become a cultural norm: that cereal for breakfast is good for you.

Twenty participants were recruited, both men and women. None of them had been diagnosed with type 2 diabetes: their fasting glucose (as measured once a year by their doctor) was in the normal range. They arrived on a weekday morning at the lab to take part in the experiment—which consisted of eating a bowl of cornflakes with milk while wearing a continuous glucose monitor.

The results of this study were alarming. In those healthy individuals, a bowl of cereal sent their glucose levels into a zone of deregulation thought to be attainable only by people with diabetes. Sixteen of the 20 participants experienced a glucose spike above 140 mg/dL (the cutoff for prediabetes, signaling problems with glucose regulation), and some even spiked above 200 mg/dL (in the range of type 2 diabetes). That didn't mean that the participants were diabetic—they weren't. But it did mean that healthy people could spike as high as diabetics and suffer the harmful side effects those spikes cause. The discovery was groundbreaking.

The fact that a bowl of cereal causes spikes makes empirical sense. Cereal is made of either refined corn or refined wheat kernels, superheated, then rolled flat or puffed into various shapes. It's pure starch, with no fiber left. And because starch is not the most palatable thing on its own, table sugar (sucrose, made of glucose and fructose) is added to the concoction. Vitamins and minerals join the mix, but the benefit of these doesn't outweigh any of the harm of the other components.

In all, 2.7 billion boxes of cereal are sold every year in the United States alone. The most popular brand is Honey Nut Cheerios, which contains three times as much sugar as the cereal used in the Stanford study. So the alarming results those researchers observed are likely conservative compared to the glucose spikes taking place in the population at large.

When 60 million Americans eat a cereal such as Honey Nut Cheerios for breakfast *every day*, 60 million Americans are pushing their glucose, fructose, and insulin levels into damaging ranges every morning. Sixty million Americans are generating swarms of free radicals in their bodies, taxing their pancreas, inflaming their cells, increasing their fat storage, and setting themselves up for a day full of cravings from shortly after they get out of bed.

Honestly, it's not their fault. Cereal is cheap, tasty, and easy to reach for while still half-asleep. My mom did it every day for a long time.

Cereal looks harmless, but it's not. That goes for granola, too.

Because of the way we eat today, early-morning spikes seem to be the norm. Whether it's cereal, toast and jam, croissants, granola, pastries, sweet oats, biscuits, fruit juice, Pop-Tarts, fruit smoothies, acai bowls, or banana bread, the typical breakfast in Western countries is composed of mostly starch and sugar: a ton of glucose and fructose.

It's a common assumption that eating something sweet for

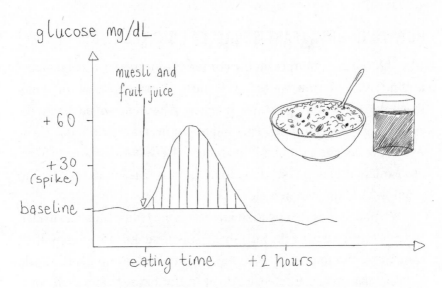

In the United States, the typical breakfast is a bowl of cereal and fruit juice. Big spike.

breakfast is a good thing because it will *give us energy.* That's what I thought, growing up, when I spread Nutella on a crepe each morning. But that's actually not correct: though eating something sweet will give us *pleasure,* it's not the best way to give us *energy.*

Why? Well, as you know, when we eat glucose, we trigger insulin production. Insulin wants to protect us from the onslaught of glucose, so it removes it from circulation. So instead of the newly digested molecules staying around in our system to be used for fuel, they are stored away—as glycogen or fat.

Scientific experiments confirm this: if you compare two diets, the one with more carbohydrates leads to less available circulating energy postdigestion. More carbs for breakfast means *less* available energy.

And that's not all I'm going to debunk here. You know the saying "Breakfast is the most important meal of the day"? It's true, but not in the way you might think.

HOW YOUR BREAKFAST SECRETLY CONTROLS YOU

If we hit our foot sharply on the corner of our dresser while dancing around our bedroom, we feel it. It hurts. (I once broke a toe doing that.) We ice it, wrap it, yet still, it may well swell up so much that we can't wear our usual shoes. That might put us in a bad mood.

If a colleague or a family member asks us "What's wrong?" we can explain it plainly: I hurt my toe this morning, and that's why I'm grumpy. The connection is clear.

When it comes to how food affects us, the connection is murkier. We don't instantly *feel* the hurt that a spiky breakfast has on us. If, as soon as we ate that bowl of cereal, we were to have a panic attack, then fall asleep at the table, we'd get it. But because metabolic processes take hours to unfold, compound over time, and become mixed with all the other things that happen in a day, connecting the dots takes a bit of detective work—at least until we get the hang of it.

A breakfast that creates a big glucose spike will make us hungry again sooner. What's more, that breakfast will deregulate our glucose levels for the rest of the day, so our lunch and dinner will also create big spikes. This is why a spiky breakfast is a one-way ticket to the glucose roller coaster. A flat breakfast, on the other hand, will make our lunch and dinner steadier.

On top of that, first thing in the morning, when we are in our fasted state, our bodies are the most sensitive to glucose. Our sink (or stomach) is empty, so anything that lands in it will be digested extremely quickly. That's why eating sugars and starches at breakfast often leads to the biggest spike of the day.

Breakfast is the *worst time* to eat just sugar and starches, yet it's the time at which most of us eat *just* sugar and starches. (It's much better to have sugar as a dessert *after* a meal, and I'll tell you more in hack 6, "Pick dessert over a sweet snack.")

TRY THIS: Write down your typical breakfast ingredients. Which ones are starches? Which are sugars? Are you eating just sugars and starches for breakfast?

I USUALLY EAT . . .	SUGARS	STARCHES	PROTEIN, FAT, OR FIBER
Example: *orange juice*	√		
Example: *oats*		√	
Example: *butter*			√

Through speaking with people who've changed their diet to keep their glucose levels steadier, I have learned that this breakfast hack is key. Choose your breakfast well, and you'll feel better throughout that day—more energy, curbed cravings, better mood, clearer skin, and on and on. Instead of feeling as though you're on the glucose roller coaster, you'll be in the driver's seat. It took a little while for Olivia to discover this, but once she did, there was no turning back.

GOOD SUGAR, BAD SUGAR, AND OLIVIA

Symptoms of dysregulated glucose can impact us at any age. Olivia, 18, from a village near Buenos Aires, Argentina, was already experiencing an assortment of them: cravings for sweets (such as dulce de leche), bad acne on her forehead, anxiety, feeling drained in the evening but unable to fall asleep.

Olivia had gone vegetarian two years before, at 16, to reduce her carbon footprint. Unfortunately, as I explained earlier, the fact that a plate of food is vegetarian (or vegan or gluten-free or organic) does not mean that it's good for you. All of us, regardless of our diet, should also think about our glucose levels.

When she talked about her symptoms with friends, they told her she should eat something healthier in the morning, something with vitamins in it. They suggested a fruit smoothie to replace her usual toast spread with jam and mug of hot chocolate. They explained to her that there was "bad sugar," from chocolate, and "good sugar," from fruit.

Olivia listened. Soon she started each morning with a fruit smoothie she blitzed at home — banana, apple, mango, kiwi.

Many people believe that some sources of sugar (namely fruits) are good for us while others — the refined sugars in sweets, cakes, and confectionary — are bad for us.

Indeed, we've been indoctrinated with the idea. A century ago, the California Fruit Growers Exchange (which represents orange producers in the United States), which later became Sunkist, created a national campaign promoting the consumption of a daily dose of orange juice for its "health giving vitamins and rare salts and acids." But it forgot to mention that fruit juice is very bad for us and we can get vitamins and antioxidants in dozens of other foods that don't hurt us in the process.

Unfortunately for Olivia, her friends had fallen for the same story. They thought that anything made from fruit was a healthy option.

To think that is to misunderstand the nature of sugar — because sugar is sugar; it's the same whether it comes from corn or beets and has been crystallized into white powder, which is how table sugar is made, or from oranges and kept in liquid form, which is how fruit juice is made. Regardless of which plant they come from, glucose and fructose molecules have the same effect on us. And denying that fruit juice is harmful *because of the vitamins it contains* is a game of dangerous deflection.

What is true, however, is that if we are going to eat some sugar, a *whole* piece of fruit is the best vehicle for it. First, in a whole piece of fruit, sugar is found in small quantities. And you'd be hard pressed to eat three apples or three bananas in one sitting—which is how much can be found in a smoothie. Even if you did eat three apples or three bananas, you would take some time to eat them, much longer than it would take you to drink them in a smoothie. So the glucose and fructose would be digested much more slowly. Eating takes longer than drinking. Second, in a whole piece of fruit, sugar is always accompanied by fiber. As I explained earlier, fiber significantly reduces the spike caused by any sugar we eat.

By blending a piece of fruit, we pulverise the fiber into tiny particles that can't fulfill their protective duties anymore. In case you're wondering, this does not happen when we chew—our jaws are powerful, but not as powerful as a blender's metal blades going 400 rotations per second. As soon as we blend, squeeze, dry, and concentrate the sugar and remove the fiber in fruit, it hits our system fast and hard—and leads to a spike.

The more denatured a fruit is, the worse it is for us. An apple is better for us than applesauce, which is better for us than apple juice. Essentially, as soon as it's juiced, dried, candied, canned, or turned to jam, you should think of fruit as *dessert*, just as you would a slice of cake. One bottle of orange juice (whether freshly squeezed, with or without pulp) contains 24 grams of sugar—that's the concentrated sugar of three whole oranges, with none of the fiber. It's the same amount of sugar as in a can of Coca-Cola. With just one bottle of

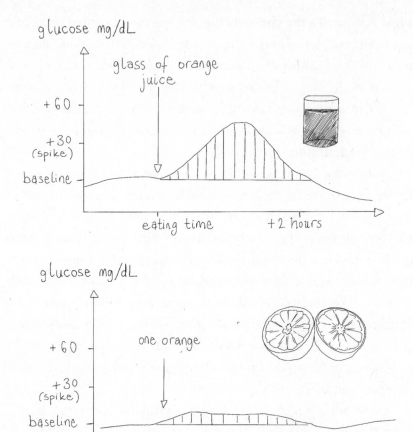

Yes, fruit juice has vitamins in it, but that's as much of a reason to drink it as the antioxidants in wine are a reason to drink alcohol.

orange juice, you've reached the limit of the number of grams of sugar you should consume in a day, according to the American Heart Association (it recommends no more than 25 grams daily for women and 36 for men).

Little wonder that with her new breakfast, things did not get better for Olivia. But she kept drinking smoothies day after day. The result? Worse acne, less energy, more anxiety, and an even harder

Most of us think that a fruit smoothie is healthier
than a breakfast with a mug of hot chocolate. In reality,
when fruits are processed, they are no better than chocolate.
Smoothies can be done right if they include other ingredients
along with fruit. More on the ideal smoothie recipe on page 132.

time falling asleep at night. Why did she feel as though she was getting worse when she was trying harder than ever to do things right?

Because her smoothie was actually creating a bigger spike than
her previous breakfast had.

Olivia found the Glucose Goddess Instagram account. She recognized that she was feeling the symptoms of glucose spikes. And it was with great relief that she learned that what she thought was a smart choice—her fruit smoothie—was actually not.

What did she do? She went savory.

GO SAVORY

The best thing you can do to flatten your glucose curves is to eat a savory breakfast. In fact, most countries have a savory option: in Japan, salad is often on the menu, and in Turkey, you'll find meat, veggies, and cheese; in Scotland, smoked fish; and in the United States, omelets.

This hack is so powerful that if you go savory for breakfast, you'll be able to eat sweet later in the day with few side effects—and I'll show you how in the next hacks.

Build your savory breakfast plate.

An ideal breakfast for steady glucose levels contains a good amount of protein, fiber, fat, and optional starch and fruit (ideally, eaten last).

If you're buying breakfast at a coffee shop, get an avocado toast, an egg muffin, or a ham and cheese sandwich, not a chocolate croissant or toast spread with jam.

Make sure your breakfast contains protein.

And no, this does not mean gobbling down 10 raw eggs every morning. Protein can be found in Greek yogurt, tofu, meat, cold cuts, fish, cheese, cream cheese, protein powder, nuts, nut butter, seeds, and, yes, eggs (scrambled, fried, poached, or soft-boiled).

To make a glucose-healthy breakfast, just go savory.
Two breakfasts with the same number of calories have vastly
different effects on glucose (and therefore insulin) levels.
In the top graph, a breakfast of starch and sugar leads to weight gain,
inflammation, and return of hunger shortly thereafter. A breakfast
of starch and fat (bottom graph) has none of those side effects.

Add fat.

Scramble your eggs in butter or olive oil, add slices of avocado, or add five almonds, chia seeds, or flaxseeds to your Greek yogurt. By the way, skip fat-free yogurt—it won't keep you full, and I'll explain why later. Switch to 5% regular or Greek yogurt.

Extra points for fiber.

It can be challenging to get fiber in the morning because it means eating veggies for breakfast. I don't blame you if you aren't into that. But if you can, try. I love mixing spinach into my scrambled eggs or tucking it underneath a sliced avocado on toast. Literally any vegetable, from spinach to mushrooms to tomatoes to zucchini to artichoke, sauerkraut, lentils, and lettuce will do.

Add starch or whole fruit for taste (optional).

Adding starch or whole fruit is optional. This can be oats, toast, rice, or potatoes or any whole fruit (the best option is berries).

Olivia decided to try the savory breakfast hack for herself. First thing the next day, she bought some eggs. To get some ideas of what else to put on her plate, she thought about her favorite lunch and dinner ingredients, and the result was a tasty dish: an omelet with avocado, sunflower seeds, olive oil, and a dash of sea salt. Very soon, she felt the difference in her body—she felt lighter, less bloated, healthier, and full of energy.

It wasn't just her body. It was her brain, too. Her studying (she's in her second year of design school) got sharper, and her grades got better. Scientists have tried to measure how various breakfasts impact our performance on cognitive tests. And the answer to whether sugar makes your brain work better is . . . no. A review of thirty-eight studies couldn't draw any definitive conclusions but stated that, if

glucose mg/dL

+60

+30
(spike)

baseline

banana, apple,
mango, kiwi
smoothie

eating time   +2 hours

glucose mg/dL

+60

+30
(spike)

baseline

omelet and
avocado

eating time   +2 hours

**The tradition that breakfast should be sweet
is completely misguided. Build your breakfast around
protein, fat, and fiber for satiety and stable energy.**

anything, a breakfast with a flatter curve could improve cognitive performance.

Furthermore, the curve created by your first meal of the day influences how the rest of the day will go. With no spike, you'll ride into the afternoon with satiety and stable energy, as Olivia learned to do. With a big spike, you'll set off a chain reaction of cravings, hunger, and lagging energy until the evening. And these chain reactions compound day after day. So if you want to improve just one aspect of your daily food habits, eat a glucose-healthy breakfast for maximum impact. You'll notice the effects immediately.

Really, it's one of the most practical changes to make. You can plan ahead. Your willpower is at its best in the morning. And there are usually no people around to encourage you to abandon it. I promise, a glucose-healthy breakfast can be as easy to put together as a bowl of cereal.

THE 5-MINUTE SAVORY BREAKFAST

(you can mix and match any of these)

No cooking involved

A bagel with cream cheese, topped with a few lettuce leaves and slices of turkey

A can of tuna, a few pecans and olives, a drizzle of olive oil

An apple with walnuts and slices of cheddar

Full-fat yogurt with sliced fruit such as a peach, a drizzle of tahini, and salt

Greek yogurt swirled with 2 tablespoons of nut butter and a handful of berries

Half an avocado with three tablespoons of hummus, lemon juice, olive oil, and salt

Homemade granola that is nut-centric or cereal designed specifically with extra fiber or protein (see the Cheat Sheets starting on page 205 to learn how to decipher packaging)

Slices of ham on crackers

Slices of smoked salmon, avocado, and tomato

Toast with almond butter

Toast with mashed avocado

Tomato and mozzarella with a drizzle of olive oil

My go-to: leftovers from last night's dinner! (the fastest option of them all!)

Cooking involved

A tortilla filled with black beans and chopped avocado

A full English breakfast (eggs, sausage, bacon, beans, tomatoes, mushrooms, toast)

Hard-boiled eggs with hot sauce and avocado

Pan-fried halloumi cheese, tomatoes, salad

Poached eggs with a side of sautéed greens

Quinoa porridge topped with a fried egg

Sausage and broiled tomatoes

Scrambled eggs with crumbled goat cheese

Toast topped with a fried egg

Warm lentils topped with a fried egg

THE STILL-SWEET BREAKFAST

If you're not ready to say goodbye to a sweet breakfast (or if you're staying with a particularly pushy aunt who likes to make pancakes from scratch in the morning), here's what to do: eat the sweet things *after* something savory.

First, eat protein, fats, and fiber—an egg, for example, a couple of spoonfuls of full-fat yogurt, or any combination of the foods from "The 5-Minute Savory Breakfast" section above and on the previous page. *Then* have the sweet food: cereal, chocolate, French toast, granola, honey, jam, maple syrup, pastries, pancakes, sugar, sweetened coffee drinks. For example, if I really want some chocolate when I wake up (What? It happens), I have it *after* a plate of eggs and spinach.

Remember the sink analogy of hack 1, "Eat foods in the right order"? With a stomach that contains other things, the impact of that chocolate or sugar and starch will be lessened.

SWEET BREAKFAST CHEAT SHEET

Can't go without something sweet in the morning? Here are some ways to eat that something but reduce its spike.

Oats

If you love oats (which are starch), eat them alongside nut butter, protein powder, yogurt, seeds, and berries. Avoid adding brown sugar, maple syrup, honey, tropical fruits, or dried fruit.

You can try a chia pudding instead: chia seeds soaked overnight in unsweetened coconut milk with a spoonful of coconut butter.

Acai bowls

Acai bowls—traditionally a Brazilian dish but now eaten around the world—are essentially a thick berry smoothie topped with granola, fruit, and other ingredients. They sound healthy because they are made from fruit, but now you know that that in no way makes something healthy. On a closer look you'll find that they are composed entirely of sugars and starches. So apply the same guidelines as for oats, above.

If you are wondering about agave and honey and how they compare to low-calorie sweeteners, we'll cover it next in hack 5, "Have any type of sugar you like—they're all the same."

Smoothies

You *can* enjoy a smoothie for breakfast; it just has to incorporate protein, fat, and fiber. Start your smoothie with protein powder, then add a combination of linseed or flaxseed oil, coconut oil, avocado, seeds, nuts, and a cup of spinach. Finally, add some sugar for taste: ideally berries, which add a sweet taste but are significantly higher in fiber than other fruits. My go-to smoothie recipe is 2 scoops of protein powder, 1 tablespoon flaxseed oil, ¼ avocado, 1 tablespoon crunchy almond butter, ¼ banana, 1 cup frozen berries, and some unsweetened almond milk.

The more protein, fat, and fiber and the less fruit your smoothie contains, the better it will be for your glucose levels.

A good rule of thumb for a smoothie: don't put more fruit into the blender than you could eat whole in one sitting.

Cereal and granola

Some cereals are better for your glucose levels than others. Look for those that brag about their high fiber content and low sugar content.

(In the Cheat Sheets included at the end of this book, I'll explain how to decipher nutrition labels on packaging to pick the best possible cereal.) Then eat it with 5% Greek yogurt instead of milk, which adds fat to the mix. Top with nuts, hemp seeds, and/or chia seeds to add protein to the mix. If you need to sweeten it, do so with berries—not sugar.

Granola may seem healthier, but it's usually just as full of sugar as cereal is. If you love it, look for a low-sugar granola with a high nut and seed content—or, even better, make your own.

Fruit

The best options to keep your glucose levels steady are berries, citrus fruits, and small, tart apples, because they contain the most fiber and smallest amount of sugar. The worst options—because they have the highest amount of sugar—are mangoes, pineapple, and other tropical fruit. Make sure you eat something else before them.

Coffee

Beware of sweetened coffee drinks—and know that cappuccinos are better for your glucose levels than mochas, which contain chocolate and sugar. If you like to have a sweetened coffee drink, try mixing the coffee with full-fat milk or cream (fat is not to be feared) and sprinkling cocoa powder on top instead. Nondairy almond or other nut milks work, too, but oat milk tends to be the biggest spiker, because it contains more carbs than the other milks, as it's made from grains, not nuts. If you add sugar to your coffee, make sure you eat something glucose-steady beforehand—even just a slice of cheese. And if you're wondering if certain sweeteners are preferable to others, read on.

What if I don't eat breakfast?

No problem. The same concept applies—whenever the first meal of your day is, make it savory to set yourself up for success.

Sweetened coffee drinks can drive a big spike.
Opt for cappuccinos, Americanos, macchiatos, and unsweetened
lattes over coffees with flavors, syrups—and sugar.

Should I try to eat my breakfast ingredients in the right order, too, as specified in hack 1?

Ideally, yes, but don't stress if you can't. The hacks in this book should be used when it's easy. If it's a bowl of full-fat yogurt topped with a seed- and nut-filled granola and you want to eat those components

together, go for it. You're already making a good choice by choosing
that over cereal.

Aren't eggs bad for your heart?

Scientists used to think that eating foods that contain cholesterol
(such as eggs) increased our risk of heart disease. Now we know
that's not true—as we learned in part 2, sugar is actually the bad guy.
Research shows that when people with type 2 diabetes replace their
oatmeal with eggs at breakfast (and keep their calories constant),
their inflammation and risk of heart disease go down.

> **TRY THIS**: Treat your breakfast like your lunch, and eat a savory
> meal. What happens? How do you feel?

LET'S RECAP

Eating cereal in the morning has become a habit for many of us,
but as you've learned in these pages, a sweet breakfast is a ticket to
a glucose roller coaster. Eating a savory one will help curb hunger,
banish cravings, boost energy, sharpen mental clarity, and more for
the next 12 hours.

Cereal for breakfast is just one of the habits I'm here to debunk.
The next one has to do with adding sugar, honey, and sweeteners
to our food and drinks—and the fact that the common assumption
about which is "healthiest" is wrong.

HAVE ANY TYPE OF SUGAR YOU LIKE— THEY'RE ALL THE SAME

You know that famous line from *Romeo and Juliet*, "A rose by any other name would smell as sweet"? Well, you could say the same thing about sugar. Sugar by any other name still has the same impact on our body.

Is honey healthier than sugar?

As you learned in hack 3, "Stop counting calories," when it comes to understanding what a food does to our bodies, it is the molecules that matter, not the calories. There is something else that doesn't matter: the *name* of the food.

This is surprising to most people, but on a molecular level, there is no difference between table sugar and honey. And there is no difference between table sugar and agave syrup. In fact, there is no difference between table sugar and any of these: agave syrup, brown sugar, caster sugar, coconut sugar, confectioner's sugar, demerara sugar, evaporated cane juice, honey, muscovado sugar, maple syrup, molasses, palm sugar, palmyra tree sugar, turbinado (raw) sugar. They are all made of glucose and fructose molecules. They are just packaged differently, named differently, and priced differently.

Honey begins as nectar from plants, but it contains glucose and fructose, just as table sugar does. Brown sugar (which sounds healthy, right?) is made of the exact same thing as white sugar, except that it is tinted (yes, *tinted*) with molasses, a by-product of the sugar-making process, to make it look more wholesome.

Muscovado sugar is even darker than brown sugar because it has even more molasses in it. Caster sugar and confectioner's sugar are table sugar ground into a finer powder. Demerara, turbinado (raw), and cane sugar are golden in color because they have been bleached less during the refinement process. Coconut sugar is sugar from a coconut instead of from a cane or a beet. Palm (or palmyra tree) sugar is from a palm. The list goes on. And misinformation is rampant: for instance, the Philippines, a large producer of coconut sugar, released data claiming that coconut sugar was healthier than regular sugar, and that was later proven to be wrong.

You get it: any kind of sugar, regardless of its color, taste, or plant of origin, is still glucose and fructose, and will still lead to glucose and fructose spikes in our bodies.

Is natural sugar better?

Many of us have heard that honey and agave contain "natural" sugars. And that dried fruit, such as dried mango, contains "natural" sugars because it comes from a fruit.

It's, um, *natural* to think that those options are better for us than table sugar. But here's something to chew on: all sugar is natural, because it always comes from a plant. Some table sugar even comes from a *vegetable* (sugar beets). But that doesn't make it any different. There is no good or bad sugar; all sugar is the same, regardless of the plant it comes from.

The molecules are what matter: by the time they reach your small intestine, they're all just glucose and fructose. Your body doesn't process sugar differently whether it came from a sugar beet, an agave plant, or a mango. As soon as a fruit is denatured and processed and its fiber is extracted, it becomes sugar like any other sugar.

glucose mg/dL

+ 60 -

+ 30 -
(spike)

baseline -

cup of coffee
with 2 tsp
brown sugar

eating time   + 2 hours

glucose mg/dL

+ 60 -

+ 30 -
(spike)

baseline -

cup of coffee
with 2 tsp
white sugar

eating time   + 2 hours

Many of us believe that brown sugar is better for us than white sugar. There is actually no difference.

It is true that in dried fruit, there is still some fiber present. But because all the water is taken out of the fruit, we eat many, many more pieces of dried fruit than we would pieces of whole fruit. So we consume way more sugar way more quickly than nature intended—and the result is big glucose and fructose spikes.

glucose mg/dL

5 Medjool dates

+ 60

+ 30 (spike)

baseline

eating time   +2 hours

Sugar is sugar. Dried fruit, such as dates, have highly concentrated amounts of sugar, and they create big, unhealthy glucose spikes. Choose whole fruits over dried fruit.

MEET AMANDA

Amanda is in her late twenties, a self-described "health nut" who watches what she eats and loves working out regularly—and continued doing so well into her first pregnancy. That was why her gestational diabetes diagnosis came as a shock. She was scared, for both herself and her baby—and she also felt judged by her friends and family. They couldn't believe her diagnosis, either. *What, you? We thought you were healthy! How's that possible?*

As the months progressed toward her due date, her glucose levels kept rising, and her insulin resistance got worse. She felt out of control. And she really thought she was eating healthily—including lots of dried fruit to satisfy her sugar cravings.

She wrote to me that the information she had found on the Glucose Goddess Instagram account had helped her take back a little bit of control. She realized that the diagnosis was not her fault. The posts and information she read there helped her see that gestational

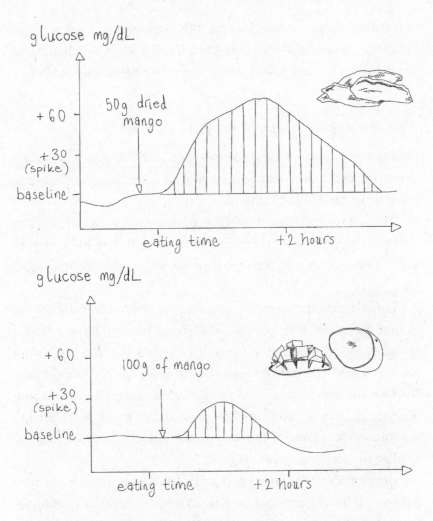

Dried fruit may seem healthy, but it's not. Dried fruit contains some fiber, but it mostly has the same molecules as table sugar: the concentrated glucose and fructose contained there hit our body like a tidal wave.

diabetes happens to many healthy people. She learned about things she could do to flatten her glucose curves and avoid going on medication.

So she quit eating the dried fruit she used to eat every day. Then she went savory for breakfast, swapping oats for eggs. Those small modifications helped her manage her gestational diabetes so well that she maintained a healthy weight throughout her pregnancy and didn't have to go on medication. I was thrilled when she shared that her baby boy arrived, and that they were both happy and healthy.

What about agave syrup's "lower glycemic index"?

During her pregnancy, Amanda was also told that agave syrup was better for her than sugar because it had a lower glycemic index. What's that about? Let's dive in.

Though sugar is sugar, regardless of its source, what *is* true is that the ratio of glucose and fructose molecules is different from sugar to sugar. Some sugars contain more fructose, while others contain more glucose.

For instance, agave syrup is often recommended to diabetics and women diagnosed with gestational diabetes because it has a "lower glycemic index" than table sugar. This is true—it does spike our glucose levels less. But the reason for this is that it contains more fructose and less glucose than regular table sugar. (Agave is about 80 percent fructose, compared to table sugar, which is 50 percent fructose.) And although this means the glucose spike it causes is smaller, the fructose spike is bigger.

Now, get this: recall from part 1 that fructose is worse for us than glucose—it overwhelms our liver, turns to fat, precipitates insulin resistance, makes us gain more weight than glucose, and doesn't make us feel as full. As a result, since agave has more fructose than table sugar does, it is actually *worse* for our health than table sugar.

Don't believe the hype.

But what about the antioxidants in honey?

This is (essentially) the same question as if we were to ask "What about the vitamins in fruit juice?" and the answer is the same: there is no logic to eating honey *for the antioxidants*, just as there's no logic to drinking fruit juice *for the vitamins*. Yes, honey contains antioxidants and fruit juice contains vitamins, but those don't outweigh the impact of the large amounts of glucose and fructose they contain. And fun fact, there aren't that many antioxidants in honey anyway; you can find all the antioxidants contained in a teaspoon of honey in *half a blueberry*. That's right—half a blueberry!

THE GOOD NEWS: PICK ANY SUGAR YOU LIKE

We don't need to eat sugar to live (recall that our body doesn't need fructose, just glucose, and it can make that from within if we don't eat it), and we don't need to eat sugar to get energy (remember, sugar actually *dampens* our energy levels).

Since all sugars, regardless of their source, are eaten for pleasure, pick whichever one you like best—and enjoy it in moderation. If you prefer the taste of honey over table sugar, go for it. If you prefer baking with brown sugar, fine too.

AND AS MUCH AS YOU CAN, CHOOSE FRUIT FOR YOUR SWEET FIX

When we want something sweet, the best thing we can do is to eat whole fruit. Remember, that's the way nature intended us to consume glucose and fructose—in small quantities, not too concentrated, in combination with fiber.

Have sliced apple in your oatmeal instead of table sugar, berries in your yogurt instead of honey.

Other ingenious additions to either oatmeal or yogurt include cinnamon, cacao powder, cacao nibs, shredded unsweetened coconut, or unsweetened nut butter (I know it sounds strange, but nut butter tastes sweet and makes for a dessert-worthy combo).

A 5% Greek yogurt with blueberries is as sweet as, but so much better for your glucose curve than, a 0% regular yogurt with honey.

ARTIFICIAL SWEETENERS

That's "natural" sugars. What about artificial sweeteners?

 Some artificial sweeteners spike our insulin levels, which mean they prime our body to store fat, encouraging weight gain. For instance, research shows that when people switch from drinking diet sodas to drinking water, they lose more weight (two extra pounds in six months in one study)—without altering the number of calories they eat.

What's more, preliminary studies suggest that the taste of sweeteners may increase our craving for sweet foods, just as sugar does.

Sugar-free Red Bull contains aspartame. Aspartame may create an insulin spike, though science doesn't yet have a definite answer. The aspartame could explain why I saw a dip in my glucose levels after drinking it—a surge in insulin leads to a drop in glucose.

The theory posits further that we could then be more likely to satisfy those cravings because sweeteners have lower calorie counts, so we think it's okay to eat another cookie. Artificial sweeteners may also change the composition of our intestinal bacteria, which could potentially have negative consequences.

The best sweeteners that have no side effects on glucose and insulin levels are:

- Allulose
- Monk fruit
- Stevia (look for pure stevia *extract* because some other forms of it are mixed with glucose-spiking fillers)
- Erythritol

There are some artificial sweeteners I'd recommend you avoid, because they are known to increase insulin and/or glucose levels, especially when combined with foods, or cause other health issues. They are:

- Aspartame
- Maltitol (turns to glucose when digested)
- Sucralose
- Xylitol
- Acesulfame-K

Sweeteners aren't a perfect replacement for sugar. Many people don't like their taste, and some even get a headache or stomachache from them. And really, they don't taste as good as sugar. Monk fruit in a breakfast shake is okay, but sometimes you just need the real stuff—when baking, for example.

The best thing to do, in my opinion, is to use sweeteners to wean ourselves off the need to sweeten everything. Because sweetness is addictive.

What about diet soda?

Let's be clear: in a vacuum, it's better to drink artificially sweetened diet soda than regular soda. *But* diet soda isn't the same as water. It contains artificial sweeteners, which can lead to some of the harmful outcomes I describe above.

THE ADDICTION CONUNDRUM

It's easy to feel addicted to eating sweet things. I once felt addicted to sweet things, too. This feeling is not our fault—remember, sweetness activates the addiction center in our brain. The more we eat it, the more we want it.

To slowly wean yourself off the taste, there are a few things you can do. Replace that spoonful of sugar in your coffee with allulose, then lower the quantity over time. Next time you want candy, try eating an apple. Or when a craving hits, notice it and take some deep breaths. In my experience, it usually passes after 20 minutes. But if you're still in the throes of it, try eating something else—usually something with fat, like cheese, does the trick. I also like drinking teas that are naturally sweet, such as cinnamon or licorice. It always helps me.

And if you still want that sweet something, eating it without guilt is the best thing to do.

LET'S RECAP

It's very unlikely that we're going to get rid of sugar in our diets entirely. And I'm here to tell you that that's okay. A birthday isn't much fun if you serve brussel sprouts instead of birthday cake.

What if, instead of trying so hard to resist it, we were to be thoughtful about when we eat it and accept—joyfully—that it's part of our lives?

I eat sugar when my mom makes birthday cake (chocolate cake with a crackly, shiny, sugary crust), when my grandmother makes *brigadeiro* (a delicious Brazilian dessert made from chocolate and sweetened condensed milk), when I eat my favorite ice cream (Häagen-Dazs Belgian chocolate topped with two spoonfuls of chocolate fudge), or when I'm craving a piece of chocolate (can you guess I like chocolate by now?). The rest of the time, if I want something sweet, I eat berries, monk fruit, almond butter, or cacao nibs.

I'm often asked questions such as "I have honey and milk before I go to bed. Is that okay?" or "Is it bad to add maple syrup when I eat pancakes?" To which I answer: Eat it if you really love it and it's worth the corresponding glucose spike.

SUGAR IS OKAY IN MODERATION

We should also try to let go of the impossible-to-keep promises we make to ourselves. I've said things such as "Starting tomorrow, I'm never eating any cupcakes ever again." Or "This is the last piece of chocolate I will buy." When we make foods off limits in an effort to force a lifestyle change, it doesn't work. The hour comes when we can't take it any longer and we empty the cookie jar.

We often think that if we can't do something perfectly, such as stick to a diet, we shouldn't do it at all. That couldn't be further from the truth. It's about trying your best.

As you start to feel better, your cravings will dissipate and you will impress yourself with how easily your sugar intake will diminish.

I promised you in the previous chapter that if you skip sugar at breakfast, I'll show you how to enjoy it later in the day. The next three hacks tell you how—in ways that will keep your glucose curves steady. That means you get to eat what you love without gaining as much weight, deepening your wrinkles, adding plaque to your arteries, or any of the other short- or long-term consequences of high glucose levels. It sounds like magic, but it's science.

HACK 6   PICK DESSERT OVER A SWEET SNACK

After a meal, we tend to move on quickly to our next activity—maybe doing the dishes, getting back to work, or going about our day. But when we're done eating, our organs are just getting started—and they keep working for *four hours* on average after our last bite. This busy time is the "posteating," or *postprandial*, state.

What happens in the postprandial state?

The postprandial state is the period of our day when the largest hormonal and inflammatory changes take place. To digest, sort, and store the molecules from the food we just consumed, blood rushes to our digestive system, our hormones rise like a tide, some systems can be put on hold (including your immune system), while others are activated (such as fat storage). Insulin levels, oxidative stress, and inflammation increase. The bigger a glucose or fructose spike after a meal, the more demanding the postprandial state is for our body to deal with because the more free radicals, glycation, and insulin release it has to manage.

The postprandial state is normal, but it's also an effort for our body. Processing a meal can take more or less effort depending on the amount of glucose and fructose we've just consumed. We tend to spend about 20 hours of a 24-hour day in the postprandial state, because we have on average three meals and two snacks a day. This used to be different: up through the 1980s, people didn't snack as often between meals, so they spent only 8 to 12 hours in the postprandial state. Snacking is a 1990s invention, like low-waisted jeans (something to think about).

When our body is not in the postprandial state, things are a little easier. Our organs are on cleanup duty, replacing damaged cells with new ones and clearing our systems. For instance, the gurgling we feel in our small intestine when we haven't eaten in a few hours is our empty digestive tract cleaning its walls. When our body is not in the postprandial state, our insulin levels come down and we can go back to burning fat instead of stashing it.

You might have heard that back in prehistoric times, we could, if needed, go a long time without eating. It's because we could easily switch between using glucose for fuel (from our last meal) to using fat for fuel (from our fat storage). This switching ability, as mentioned earlier, is called *metabolic flexibility*. It is a prime measure of a healthy metabolism.

Remember Marie, who used to leave the house with a purse full of snacks? She was an example of low metabolic flexibility. She *needed* to eat every 90 minutes because her cells had come to rely on glucose for fuel every few hours. When Marie changed the way she ate, she retrained her cells to use fat for fuel instead. She could then go hours without eating. Marie increased her metabolic flexibility.

To increase your own metabolic flexibility, eat larger, more filling meals so you don't need to snack every hour or two. That goes against a popular belief that eating "six small meals a day" is better than two or three big ones, but research bears it out. Scientists in the Czech Republic, in 2014, tested this in people with type 2 diabetes. They decided on a daily calorie quota and got one group of participants to consume their calories in two large meals and the other group to consume them in six small meals. The two-meal group not only lost more weight (8 pounds versus 5 pounds in three months) but saw improvements in the key markers of their overall health: their fasting glucose decreased, their liver fat decreased, their insulin resistance decreased, and their pancreas cells got healthier. Same

**Same pineapple, different spike. If it's eaten as a dessert after
a meal containing fat, fiber, and protein, pineapple will create a smaller
spike. We do see a small reactive hypoglycemia, but this is less of
an issue than the big spike when pineapple is eaten as a snack.
Bigger spike, more symptoms.**

calories, different effects. (Back to one of my favorite topics: calories
aren't everything.)

Another way to improve your metabolic health is via what's
called *intermittent fasting*, where you either fast for 6, 9, 12, or

16 hours at a time or drastically reduce your calorie intake a couple of days a week. But this chapter is not about that. This chapter is about an insight from the latest research on glucose spikes: if you want to eat something sweet, it's better to have it as dessert rather than as a snack in the middle of the day on an empty stomach. Understanding the postprandial state is key to learning why.

WHY DESSERT WINS

When we forgo snacks, we keep our system out of the postprandial state for longer. That means there's time for the cleanup I described above. And by eating something sweet after a meal, we lessen the corresponding glucose spike it would cause because—shout-out to hack 1—eating sugar and starches *last*, after other food (instead of first, or on their own as a snack), means they move from sink to pipe more slowly.

So whether it's a piece of fruit, a smoothie, a candy bar, or a cookie, if you're going to eat it, do it at the end of a meal.

> **TRY THIS:** If you feel the urge to eat something sweet between meals, put it aside—in the fridge or somewhere else—and enjoy it for dessert after your next meal instead.

MEET GHADEER

Ghadeer is a translator and mother of three who lives in Kuwait. She suffers from PCOS and has done so since her first period, at 13. She has contended with all its symptoms, from acne to mood swings to weight gain. She has experienced several miscarriages. A few years ago, at 31 years old, she was diagnosed with insulin resistance and her period stopped altogether.

glucose mg/dL

fruit smoothie on an empty stomach

+60

+30 (spike)

baseline

eating time   +2 hours

glucose mg/dL

fruit smoothie after lunch

+60

+30 (spike)

baseline

eating time   +2 hours

It's all about reducing glucose fluctuations. Jamba Juice on an empty stomach created a spike of about 50 mg/dL; after a meal, the overall variability it caused was lower.

Her doctor encouraged her to change her lifestyle—to eat better and exercise more. But she was lost as to where to begin. It was pretty vague advice, as advice goes, and was received without much enthusiasm. Ghadeer didn't understand what to do next, nor did she believe that what she did could manage her condition—until the day she came across the Glucose Goddess Instagram account.

There, it all clicked. Insulin resistance and PCOS are linked. Both have the same cause—dysregulated glucose levels. That information changed Ghadeer's life. On top of that, she was thrilled when she realized she could address her symptoms without going on yet another diet. She had been on what felt like a hundred diets—and she was tired of diets. She never wanted to go on one ever again.

So she tried a few of these hacks. She started to eat her food in the right order. She swapped fruit juice for tea. She replaced sugar for monk fruit. She didn't stop eating chocolate and candy, which she loves, but she now eats them as dessert instead of as snacks. Her days now consist of three meals instead of three meals plus snacks.

In three months, her period came back. Other changes: her average glucose level used to be 162 mg/dL; now it's 90 mg/dL. She lost over 20 pounds, and she has rid herself of PCOS symptoms and insulin resistance. She feels the difference in her mood, too: she's more patient with her kids. "I have never, in my whole life, felt like this. I feel so good. My body is my friend now."

The changes were so drastic that her doctor marveled. "What did you do?" he asked. She shared everything she had learned.

Should I try to eat only once or twice a day?

You don't need to go that far. Some people find that this form of intermittent fasting suits them very well, others that it's hard to keep up with. Studies have shown that the benefits are more pronounced for men and that for women of reproductive age, fasting too long and too often may cause hormonal disruptions and other types of biological stress. Try three meals a day, and see how you feel.

What about late-night snacking?

If you typically have a sweet snack a few hours after dinner, a better alternative is to have it as dessert after you finish your entrée. If a late-night snack is inevitable, read on for other hacks that will help.

How do I know if I'm metabolically flexible?

If you can easily go five hours between meals without feeling light-headed, shaky, or hangry, you're likely to be metabolically flexible.

LET'S RECAP

The best time to eat something sweet is after you've already eaten a meal with fat, protein, and fiber. When we eat sugar on an empty stomach, we're throwing our system into a postprandial spin, riding on a big glucose and fructose spike. But if you can't avoid eating sugar on an empty stomach—a last-minute birthday party invite, a workday bake-off, an ice cream date with your crush—I'm here for you. Read on to discover another supercool hack.

HACK 7   REACH FOR VINEGAR BEFORE YOU EAT

Do you want to drizzle some vinegar on your brownie? Didn't think so. Don't worry, that's not what I am about to suggest. I'm talking about mixing a vinegar drink and sipping it before you eat your next sweet treat—whether for dessert or on the occasions when you have it as a stand-alone snack.

The recipe is simple, but the impact is strong. A drink consisting of a tablespoon of vinegar in a tall glass of water, drunk a few minutes *before* eating something sweet, flattens the ensuing glucose and insulin spikes. With that, cravings are curbed, hunger is tamed, and more fat is burned. This is a very cheap trick, too: a standard bottle of vinegar costs under $10 at your corner store and contains over 60 1-tablespoon servings. You're welcome.

Vinegar is a sour-tasting liquid made by fermenting alcohol, thanks to common bacteria which turns it into acetic acid. These bacteria are ever present in our world—they are even in the air we breathe. If you leave a glass of wine sitting out on your table and go on vacation, when you return in a few weeks it will have turned to vinegar.

Common varieties of vinegar include rice vinegar, white wine vinegar, red wine vinegar, sherry vinegar, balsamic vinegar, and apple cider vinegar. Among all the vinegars, though, one is most popular for this hack: apple cider vinegar (ACV). The reason is that most people find that it tastes better than the other vinegars when diluted in that tall glass of water. But all vinegars work identically on our glucose, so pick the one you please. (Note that lemon juice does not have the same effect because it contains citric acid, not acetic acid.)

MEET MAHNAZ

Vinegar has been touted as a health remedy for centuries. In the eighteenth century it was even prescribed in tea form to diabetics. In Iran it's consumed many times a day, in various water-based drinks, by people of all ages. "In my family we've been drinking apple cider vinegar for generations," explained Mahnaz, a Glucose Goddess community member from Tehran. "My grandmother makes her own and distributes it to all family members. We drink it because it's part of our culture and it's been passed on that it's good for us. As to why exactly it's good for us, I had no idea until I found your account."

This is Mahnaz's grandmother's recipe, in case you want to get into fermenting, too:

> Mash clean and sweet apples.
> Put into barrels.
> Cover and leave alone for 10 to 12 months.
> The place should be hot.
> And sunlight is very good.
> Insects are okay and a sign of good vinegar.
> So don't panic, they are just helping.
> When it is ready, you should strain the liquid very well, twice,
>   using a fabric with tiny holes.

Though people have been drinking vinegar for centuries, it's only recently that scientists have been able to understand the mechanisms behind its health benefits.

In the past decade, a couple of dozen research teams around the globe have measured the effects of vinegar on our body. Here is how most of the studies went: Put together a group of 30 to a few hundred participants. Ask half the group to drink 1 or 2 tablespoons of vinegar in a tall glass of water before their meals for three months and give the other group a placebo, something that tastes like vinegar but isn't vinegar. Track their weight, blood markers, and body composition. Make sure both groups maintain identical diet and exercise, sit back, grab popcorn, and watch.

What researchers found was that by adding vinegar before meals for three months, the subjects lost two to four pounds and reduced their visceral fat, waist and hip measurements, and triglyceride levels. In one study, both groups were put on a strict weight-loss diet, and the vinegar group lost twice as much weight (11 versus 5 pounds), even though they ate the same number of calories as the nonvinegar group. A Brazilian research team explained that because of its effect on fat loss, vinegar is more effective than many thermogenic supplements touted as fat burners.

The positive effects of vinegar are many. In nondiabetics, insulin-resistant people, people with type 1 or type 2 diabetes alike, as little as 1 tablespoon a day significantly decreases glucose levels. The effects are also seen in women with PCOS: in a tiny study (which definitely needs replication before it's confirmed), four out of seven women got their periods back in 40 days when they added one vinegar drink a day.

Here's what happened in all these participants' bodies: when they drank vinegar before eating a meal rich in carbohydrates, the glucose spike from that meal was reduced by 8 to 30 percent.

To understand how this happens, we have an important clue: the amount of insulin also decreases when vinegar is consumed before eating (by about 20 percent in one study).

This tells us that drinking vinegar does not flatten glucose curves by increasing the amount of insulin in the body. And this is a very good thing. Indeed, you *could* flatten a glucose curve by injecting someone with insulin or giving them a medication or a drink that would release more insulin into their system. This is because the more insulin there is in the body, the more your liver, muscles, and fat cells work to remove any excess glucose from the bloodstream and quickly store it away. However, although insulin brings glucose levels down, it also increases inflammation and weight gain. What we really want to do is flatten our glucose curves *without increasing the amount of insulin in the body*. Which is what vinegar does.

So how does it work? Scientists believe that several things could be at play.

Here is a test I ran to illustrate the science: vinegar curbs a glucose spike.

HOW VINEGAR WORKS

Remember the enzyme that Jerry and humans have in common, alpha-amylase? This is the enzyme that in plants chops starch back up into glucose and in humans turns bread to glucose in our mouths. Scientists have found that the acetic acid in vinegar temporarily inactivates alpha-amylase. As a result, sugar and starch are transformed into glucose more slowly, and the glucose hits our system more softly. You may recall from hack 1, "Eat foods in the right order," that fiber also has this effect on alpha-amylase, which is one of the reasons fiber helps flatten our glucose curves, too.

Second, once acetic acid gets into the bloodstream, it penetrates our muscles: there, it encourages our muscles to make glycogen faster than they usually would, which in turn leads to more efficient uptake of glucose.

These two factors—glucose being released into the body more slowly and our muscles uptaking it more quickly—mean that there is less free-flowing glucose present, so less of a glucose spike.

What's more, acetic acid not only reduces the amount of insulin present—which helps us get back to fat-burning mode—it also has a remarkable effect on our DNA. It tells our DNA to reprogram a bit so that our mitochondria burn more fat. Yep. For real.

What does this mean for us?

This hack works for both sweet and starchy foods. Maybe you're ready to dig into a big bowl of pasta. Maybe you're about to eat the slice of cherry pie you've set aside for your dessert. Or maybe you're at a birthday party and you must have chocolate cake in the middle of the afternoon (and you're thankful they didn't serve brussel sprouts instead). Reach for vinegar first to counter some of the side effects of a glucose spike.

Grab a tall glass of water (some people find that hot water is

Any type of vinegar works. One tablespoon of rice vinegar in a bowl of white rice (as per Japanese tradition) will help steady your glucose levels.

more soothing), and pour 1 tablespoon of vinegar into it. If you don't like the taste, start with a teaspoon or even less, and build up to it. Grab a straw, down the drink either less than 20 minutes before, during the course of, or less than 20 minutes after eating the glucose-spiking food.

Here's an even easier way to use this hack: now that you're adding

There you have it: eat your ice cream, and help your body, too.

a green starter to all your meals, you can add some vinegar to your dressing. In the first ever study looking at vinegar and glucose spikes, two meals were consumed: one group ate a salad with olive oil, then bread, and the other group ate a salad with olive oil *and vinegar*, then bread. In participants who had the dressing with vinegar, the glucose spike was 31 percent smaller. So order vinaigrette instead of ranch dressing next time.

Vinegar to curb a glucose spike is most useful when it's consumed

glucose mg/dL

salad with olive oil,
then rice bowl

+ 60

+30
(spike)

baseline

eating time   + 2 hours

glucose mg/dL

salad with olive oil
and vinegar, then
rice bowl

+ 60

+30
(spike)

baseline

eating time   + 2 hours

For your green starter, the best dressing for your glucose levels incorporates vinegar—like a traditional vinaigrette.

during a meal that would otherwise cause a big spike, but really, you can use it anytime—depending on your level of commitment. (And in the next few pages, I share even more recipes for using vinegar in this way.)

To be clear: You can't vinegar yourself out of a bad diet. Vinegar curbs spikes, but doesn't erase them. It will help if you add it to your diet—but it's not a justification to eat more sugar, because on balance, that would make your diet worse than before.

BACK TO MAHNAZ

Mahnaz's mom was diagnosed with type 2 diabetes after her third pregnancy 16 years ago. It was hard for her to manage that condition, despite the family apple cider vinegar production (consuming vinegar alone will not prevent someone from getting diabetes). So Mahnaz told her about the hacks in this book. Mahnaz's mother started to eat her food in the right order and switched to savory breakfasts. She was already drinking vinegar in a tall glass of water, so she kept at it. In four months, she went from 200 mg/dL fasting glucose level to 110 mg/dL, from severely diabetic to diabetic no longer.

I mention this in part to remind you that the hacks in this book are tools in your toolbox. Some may be easier than others to incorporate into your life. Some may work better for you than others and in different combinations. But they are all beneficial. And the more of them you use, the more successful you'll be in flattening your glucose curves.

Why do I need a straw?

Even though diluted vinegar is not acidic enough to damage your teeth's enamel, I would suggest you drink it with a straw just to be safe. Never swig it straight from the bottle. As part of other foods, such as vinaigrette, it's fine.

How much time should I wait between the vinegar and the food?

Ideally, drink it 20 minutes (or less) before eating. You can also drink it *during*, or up to 20 minutes *after*, eating, and it will work almost as well.

All vinegars work. Here, white wine vinegar. The Brits had it right!

Are there any negative side effects?

You shouldn't experience any negative side effects as long as you stick to drinkable vinegar—i.e., vinegar with 5 percent acidity (cleaning vinegar has 6 percent acidity, so if it's next to the mops and toilet paper at the supermarket, don't drink it!). For some people, vinegar can irritate their mucous membranes; for others, it can cause heartburn. It's not recommended for people with stomach disorders, although that is just a precaution—no studies have been done to measure the effects. Vinegar does not appear to damage the stomach lining, since it's actually less acidic than gastric juices and even less acidic than Coca-Cola or lemon juice. Again, it's up to you—listen to your body and if vinegar doesn't agree with you, don't force it.

Is there a limit to how much I can drink?

Well, yes. A 29-year-old woman who consumed 16 tablespoons of vinegar every day for six years was admitted to the hospital because of very low levels of potassium, sodium, and bicarbonate. So don't do that. That's way too much. But most people do fine drinking a tablespoon in a tall glass of water a few times a day.

Can I have it while pregnant or breastfeeding?

Most standard vinegars are pasteurized and safe to consume. Apple cider vinegar, on the other hand, is usually unpasteurized, which may present risks to pregnant women. Check with your doctor first.

Uh-oh, I forgot to drink vinegar, and now I've eaten a slice of cake. Is it too late?

No! I do this all the time. Sometimes the slice of cake is so tasty that I forget about the precake drink. No worries. Drinking it after eating something sweet or starchy (again, up to 20 minutes after) is much better than not drinking it at all. It still has glucose-lowering effects.

How about pills and gummies?

When it comes to vinegar pills or capsules, the jury is still out. They may work as well as vinegar in liquid form, but it's not certain. If you want to try them, you might need to swallow 3 or more pills to get the amount of acetic acid in a tablespoon of vinegar (about 800 milligrams).

Gummies aren't a good move: they contain sugar (about 1 gram of sugar per gummy). So not only might they not work to flatten your glucose curves, they actually lead to spikes. (I reached out to one leading apple cider vinegar gummy brand to ask for scientific backing for its claims—I didn't get an answer.)

How about kombucha?

Kombucha has less than 1 percent acetic acid, and if it's not home-made, it often has added sugar in it. So although it is not a spike slasher, it still has some health benefits: since it's a fermented food, it contains beneficial bacteria that fuel the good microbes in our gut.

I don't like the taste of vinegar. What should I do?

Start with a small quantity, and work your way up. Try white vinegar instead of apple cider vinegar (some people prefer the taste). Or consider mixing the vinegar and water with some other ingredients—it doesn't matter what is mixed in along with it (except don't mix it with sugar, as that will negate the effects).

Here are some recipes from Glucose Goddess community members:

- A cup of hot cinnamon tea and 1 tablespoon of apple cider vinegar
- A glass of water, a pinch of salt, a pinch of cinnamon, and 1 teaspoon of apple cider vinegar
- A glass of water, a pinch of salt, 1 teaspoon of liquid aminos, and 1 tablespoon of apple cider vinegar
- A teapot of hot water, with a wedge of lemon, some ginger root, 1 tablespoon of apple cider vinegar, and a pinch

of allulose, monk fruit, stevia extract or erythritol for sweetness

- Sparkling water, ice, and 1 teaspoon of apple cider vinegar
- Vegetables fermented in a jar full of apple cider vinegar

LET'S RECAP

Adding vinegar to our diet, either in a drink or a salad dressing, is an excellent way to flatten our glucose curves. It does so in two ways: it slows the arrival of glucose into the bloodstream, then increases the speed at which our muscles soak it up and turn it into glycogen. Speaking of muscles, they seem to be pretty good at this job . . .

HACK 8　AFTER YOU EAT, MOVE

Every three to four seconds, our eyelid muscles receive a message from our brain in the form of electric signals, or *impulses*. The signals contain a simple instruction: "Blink now, please, so that we can hydrate these eyes and keep reading this amazing book." Across our entire body, muscles contract to make us walk, lean, grab, lift, and more. Some muscles we consciously control (for example, our fingers), others we don't (for example, our heart).

The more and the harder a muscle is told to contract, whether consciously or unconsciously, the more energy it needs. The more energy it needs, the more glucose it needs. (The mitochondria in muscle cells can also use other things to make energy, such as fat, but when glucose is abundant, that's the fast, ready fuel of choice.) There is a special name, by the way, for the energy created out of the ashes of glucose to fuel our cells: adenosine triphosphate, or ATP.

The rate of glucose burning varies widely depending on how hard we're working—i.e., how much ATP is required by our muscles. It can increase 1,000-fold from when we are at rest (sitting on our couch watching TV) to when we are intensely exercising (sprinting to catch our dog running across the park).

With every new muscle contraction, glucose molecules are burned up. And we can use this fact to our advantage to flatten our glucose curves.

MEET KHALED

Khaled is 45 years old. He lives in the sunny, hot United Arab Emirates, where year-round beach days are the norm. Up until recently, Khaled didn't lie out to tan when he went to the seaside—he always wore a T-shirt, he said, to hide his belly from his friends.

Change is hard, so the best shot we have at making it work is choosing strategies that require very little effort but lead to big results. (Say, like, the hacks in this book.)

Like many of us, totally understandably, Khaled had no desire to change what he ate, but he was open to other ideas. Right before the COVID-19 pandemic, he came across the Glucose Goddess Instagram account. Seeing the effect of these hacks, mapped out in graphs, ignited something inside him—not least because his father and siblings are diabetic. When lockdown set in, Khaled suddenly had a lot of time on his hands, and he decided to try something new—as long as it was easy.

He decided he'd try walking after meals, which is one of the hacks I talk about on my Instagram account. Nothing he ate had to change. He just had to stand up after his lunch of rice and meat and go for a 10-minute walk in his neighborhood.

As he walked, he imagined the glucose from the rice moving into his leg muscles, instead of heading to his fat reserves. When he got home, he surprised himself—instead of wanting to reach for sweets and then take a nap, as he usually did after lunch, he returned to his desk and worked through the afternoon. He felt . . . good. The next day, the 10 minutes of walking turned into 20. He continued on with this new habit.

There are multiple traditions that recommend walking after eating, such as the Indian custom of "100 steps after a meal," and they exist for good reason. As soon as the influx of glucose (from a large bowl of rice, for example) hits our body, two things can happen. If we stay sedentary as the spike reaches its peak, glucose floods our cells and overwhelms our mitochondria. Free radicals are produced, inflammation increases, and excess glucose is stored away in the liver, muscles, and fat.

If, on the other hand, we contract our muscles as the glucose moves from our intestine to our bloodstream, our mitochondria have a higher burning capacity. They aren't overwhelmed as quickly—they are thrilled to use the extra glucose to make ATP to fuel our

When we eat starches or sugars, we have two choices:
either stay still and let the spike happen, or move and curb the spike.

If we sit in a chair for an hour after eating cake, the glucose will accumulate in our body and cause a spike. If we exercise instead, the glucose will almost immediately be used up by our muscles. It won't accumulate and cause a spike.

working muscles. On a continuous glucose monitor graph, the difference is stark.

Here's another way to think about it: when we exercise (again, just 10 minutes of walking is helpful), we make the fire on our grandfather's steam train bigger and hotter. Our grandfather shovels coal at a greater speed; the steam train burns it at a greater speed. Instead of accumulating, the extra glucose is used up.

So we can eat the exact same thing, and then, by using our muscles afterward (within one hour and 10 minutes of eating; more on that below), flatten the glucose curve of that food.

Over the next six months, Khaled kept on walking for 20 minutes after lunch or dinner. Then he started to eat food in the right order. He lost 16 pounds. Remarkable, I know. And he's beaming. He shared, "I feel younger than ever before. When I compare myself to other people my age, I am doing way more, have more energy, and am happier. My friends ask me what I've done. . . . I'm happy to share the hacks. It's helped everyone in my family, too."

Many people, like Khaled, walk 10 to 20 minutes after meals, and they've seen excellent results. A large 2018 research review looked at 135 people with type 2 diabetes and found that aerobic exercise (walking) after eating decreased their glucose spike by up to 27 percent.

If you want to hit the gym after meals, that's going to help even more—although some people find strenuous exercise on a full stomach quite hard. The good news is, you can work out at any time up to 70 minutes after the end of your meal to curb a glucose spike; 70 minutes is around the time when that spike reaches its peak, so using your muscles before that is ideal. You can also use your muscles acutely in a push-up, a squat, a plank, or any weight-lifting exercise. Resistance exercise (weight lifting) has been shown to decrease the glucose spike by up to 30 percent and the size of further spikes over the following 24 hours by 35 percent. It's rare that you'll be able to curb the *entire* glucose spike, but you can make a sizable dent in it.

And here's the kicker: when we move after eating, we flatten our glucose curve *without increasing our insulin level*—just as was the case with vinegar. While usually our muscles need insulin to stash glucose away, if our muscles are currently contracting, they don't need insulin to be able to uptake glucose.

And the more our muscles contract and uptake glucose without needing insulin, the smaller the glucose spike will be, so the less insulin will be dispatched by the pancreas to deal with the remaining glucose. This is great news all around. Going for even just a 10-minute walk after a meal will lessen the side effects of whatever we just ate. And the longer we work out, the more our glucose and insulin curves will flatten.

WHY YOU SHOULD WATCH TV AFTER DINNER

You're home, you've had a bowl of pasta for dinner (after a green salad, right?), you're about to sit on the couch and turn on your favorite TV show. But if you're able to multitask, try doing some squats while you're watching the screen. Or try a wall sit with your back against the wall, do triceps dips off the edge of the couch, hold a side plank, or a boat pose on the carpet. A Glucose Goddess community member named Monica has a fun setup: she keeps a kettlebell behind her couch, and after eating something sweet, she sets a 20-minute timer on her phone—when it goes off, she grabs the weight and does 30 squats, holding the kettlebell.

Office variation: You have no time to go for a walk after your meal. That's okay. Go up and down the building stairs a couple of times, pretending you need to use the restroom. While in a meeting, do some quiet calf raises on the floor. Or a set of elevated push-ups against your desk. Problem solved.

TRY THIS: Rate how you feel when you have a sweet snack and then stay sitting. Rate how you feel when you have the same treat and walk 20 minutes afterward. How is your energy? How is your hunger level in the next few hours?

How quickly after eating should I exercise?

Monica gets active 20 minutes after eating, but you can exercise any-time within 70 minutes after eating to see an effect. As mentioned above, you want your muscles to start contracting before the glucose spike reaches its peak. I like to go for a walk or do strength or resis-tance exercises in front of the TV about 20 minutes after a meal. But in various studies, many different scenarios have been tested: some people started walking right after they put their fork down, some 10 to 20 minutes after finishing their meal. Others waited 45 minutes after eating to start a workout. All worked well.

Should I exercise before or after a meal?

Exercising after a meal seems to be the best option, but before is also useful. In a study of resistance training in obese people, exercising *before* dinner (eating 30 minutes after the workout was over) low-ered their glucose and insulin spikes by 18 percent and 35 percent, respectively, as opposed to 30 percent and 48 percent if the exercise was started 45 minutes *after* dinner.

How about other times during the day?

Exercising *anytime* is great for you. And it has many more positive side effects than just curbing a glucose spike. Among other things, it helps increase our mental well-being, energizes us, helps our heart stay healthy, and reduces inflammation and oxidative stress. Whether you're fasted or not, if you take up a new physical activity, your over-all glucose levels will start decreasing as you put on muscle mass.

However, if you're thinking of adding more walking to your daily regime and you can do it at any time, it'll be most impactful after meals.

How many minutes of exercise do I need?

It's up to you to find what works. Studies usually look at 10 to 20 minutes of walking or 10-minute strength or resistance sessions. I've found that I have to do about 30 squats to see any change to my glucose level.

Why does fasted exercise lead to a glucose spike? Is that bad?

When you exercise and you haven't yet eaten, i.e., you are engaging in fasted exercise, your liver releases glucose into your blood to fuel the mitochondria in your muscles. This shows up on a glucose monitor as a spike—because there is one. These spikes do cause oxidative stress, by increasing free radicals, but the exercise that causes them also increases your ability to get rid of free radicals, and, importantly, that improved defense against free radicals lingers longer than the acute, exercise-induced production of free radicals. Thus, the net effect of exercise is to reduce oxidative stress. Exercise is therefore considered a *hormetic* stress on the body. This means that it is a type of beneficial stress that causes our bodies to become more resilient.

LET'S RECAP

If you're going to eat something sweet or starchy, use your muscles afterward. Your muscles will happily uptake excess glucose as it arrives in your blood, and you'll lessen the glucose spike, reduce the likelihood of weight gain, and avoid an energy slump. Postmeal sleepiness is particularly curbed by this technique. And it works even better when you drink vinegar mixed into a tall glass of water before you eat.

Now you know the amazing combo for snacking on something sweet without incurring a big glucose spike in your body: vinegar before, exercise after.

**The more the merrier: combining hacks is incredibly powerful.
Bookending a sweet treat by drinking apple cider vinegar beforehand,
then using your muscles afterward, will help you reduce the side effects.**

IF YOU HAVE TO SNACK, GO SAVORY

I've mentioned how glucose impacts both our bodies and our minds throughout this book. Back when I embarked on this research, however, it was always easier to discern glucose's physical rather than mental effects. I knew why I saw acne on my nose or why I gained weight. Until one day—when I looked at the data from my own glucose monitor after I ate a doughnut.

Since my accident at 19, I've struggled with a mental health condition that I've named "splitting" or "feeling split." Clinically, it's called *depersonalization*. When it happens, it feels as though I partially leave my body. When I look in the mirror, I don't recognize myself. When I look down at my hands, I think they belong to someone else. A fog sets in in front of my eyes. I lose my unified sense of "I," and my mind starts to spin uncontrollably as I think about existential questions. It's very scary, especially if I'm alone.

The thing that gets me through those moments is to remember that they will pass. I've found a lot of help in talk therapy, eye movement desensitization and reprocessing, or EMDR (remembering the accident while my therapist taps on my knees alternately), and craniosacral therapy (a form of bodywork). I was lucky that I knew someone close to me who had experienced the same thing when he was younger—my cousin. I would text him whenever I needed reassurance. "I know it's awful. Trust me, it will pass," he would respond. I also turned to my diaries. I wrote a lot.

I felt split for a full year after my surgery. Then the feeling would come and go once a week or once a month and last for a few hours.

I did everything to try to find out what triggered and what resolved that feeling. But most of the time, I simply didn't know.

Then, eight years after my accident, I realized that one of the triggers could be . . . food.

In April 2018, my boyfriend and I and a couple of friends were visiting the seaside city of Kamakura on the coast of Japan. I had been wearing a glucose monitor for just about a month.

We had breakfast very early. Five hours later, we were hungry again. We stopped for coffee and doughnuts, then headed for a walk by the ocean.

As we talked about our next adventures—viewing cherry blossoms, visiting Harajuku, and more—I began to notice a shift in my mental state. The feeling was all too familiar. I knew I was about to split.

The fog set in. I looked at hands that were not my own. I knew I was speaking, but I didn't really know what I was saying or why. As is usually the case, I didn't confide in my friends, fearful that I would be a burden to them.

Through the fog, I scanned my glucose monitor. It was a habit by now; I had been doing it every few hours since I started wearing it.

The doughnuts we had eaten 30 minutes before had created the biggest glucose spike I had ever seen: from 100 mg/dL to 180 mg/dL.

I realized I had potentially found a trigger for the splitting: a very steep glucose spike. And in fact, in the ensuing months and years, I was able to prove it. When I felt split, I would recall what I had eaten that day. It happened if I had had chocolate cake for dinner instead of a normal meal or if I'd had cookies for breakfast.

Now, this is not to say that flattening my glucose curves has cured my depersonalization. I still feel split when I don't spend enough time alone, when I'm holding stress in my body, and for other reasons that I don't yet understand, and sometimes I'll experience a big

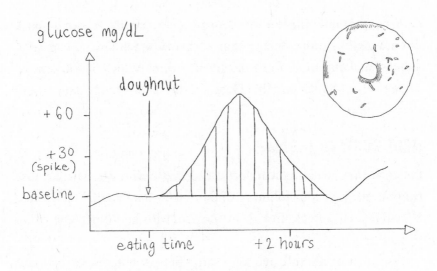

glucose mg/dL

doughnut

+60

+30
(spike)

baseline

eating time   +2 hours

The doughnut spike that made me split.

glucose spike and not feel split at all. But this new awareness has definitely helped.

I did some research and didn't find any studies showing an episode of depersonalization being triggered by food. I did discover, however, that in people with this mental health condition, some areas of the brain are more metabolically active—that is, they consume more glucose—than others. More glucose in the body, more glucose in the brain, so potentially more glucose in those hyperactive areas, too. Maybe that would cause the issue.

Certainly, we know that food affects how we feel. Science tells us that when people eat a diet that leads to lots of glucose spikes, they report worsening moods over time and more depressive symptoms compared to a diet of similar calories but with flatter curves.

Many community members have also shared that sugary foods increase their anxiety.

We all, from time to time, feel the urge to snack on something sweet—often when we're feeling sleepy. However, the idea that eating something sweet will energize us is a myth. A sweet snack doesn't give us more energy than a savory snack, and it can actually just make us more tired shortly afterward. Which, if you have to drive twelve hours a day, like Gustavo, can be positively dangerous.

MEET GUSTAVO (AGAIN)

Gustavo taught us his wonderful broccoli-before-the-steak-house tip that allowed him to enjoy dinners with his friends and flatten his curves. He's back, live from Mexico, with another piece of information.

Gustavo needs to drive long shifts between states for his sales job. He often stays 6, 8, 12 hours on the road at a time. In the old days, when he stopped at a gas station, feeling exhausted, he would pick up candy or a granola bar to "get some energy." He'd get back behind the wheel, feel energized for about 45 minutes, then exhausted once again. He was very likely not metabolically flexible: his body couldn't switch to using his fat reserves for fuel, so he needed to eat starch or sugar often. Little did he know that, as we learned in hack 4, "Flatten your breakfast curve," because of how insulin works, the glucose in a candy or granola bar tends to go to storage rather than to be used as fuel. So when we eat something sweet, there is actually *less* energy circulating in our body after digestion than when we eat something savory. Gustavo would briefly feel perked up by his snack. But it didn't last very long, and an hour later he'd be tired and have to stop for another one.

As I mentioned in hack 2, "Add a green starter to all your meals," Gustavo first decided to make lifestyle changes after people close to him passed away from complications related to type 2 diabetes. Gustavo also swapped out cereal in the morning and subbed in a glucose-steady smoothie that he makes with flaxseed, nopal (prickly pear cactus), and maca root (he says it tastes better than it sounds). Out with the sitting around after eating, in with the walking. Now it was time to smarten up his snacking when on the road: no more candy or granola bar from the gas station; much better to take some carrots, cucumber, and peanut butter with him. Which he now always does.

These days, with his flatter glucose curves, Gustavo doesn't feel the overwhelming desire to nap in the middle of the highway. His energy is steady throughout his drives. He has also lost 88 pounds, reduced his depression medication, and cleared his brain fog.

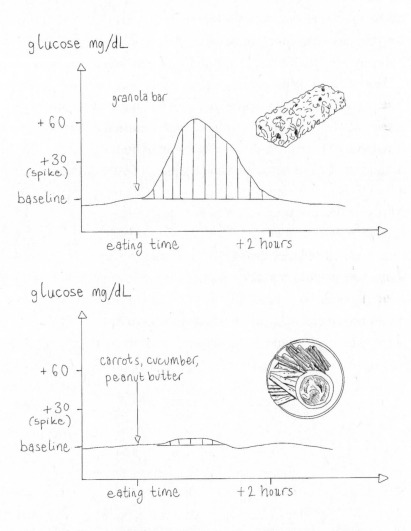

For steady energy, pick snacks that don't spike your glucose levels.

If you're looking for energy, and I know it's counterintuitive, skip the sweet snack—don't pick up candy or a granola bar. Instead, choose a savory snack. And not a starchy one, either, since starch also turns to glucose.

Here are my go-to savory snacks.

THE 30-SECOND NO-GLUCOSE-SPIKE SAVORY SNACK

Apple slices smeared with nut butter
Apple slices with a hunk of cheese
Bell pepper slices dipped in a spoonful of guacamole
Celery smeared with nut butter
A cup of 5% Greek yogurt topped with a handful of pecans
A cup of 5% Greek yogurt with nut butter swirled into it
A handful of baby carrots and a spoonful of hummus
A handful of macadamia nuts and a square of 90% dark chocolate
A handful of pork rinds
A hard-boiled egg with a dash of hot sauce
A hunk of cheese
Lightly salted coconut slivers
Seeded crackers with a slice of cheese
A slice of ham
A soft-boiled egg with a dash of salt and pepper
A spoonful of nut butter

HACK 10   PUT SOME CLOTHES ON YOUR CARBS

I don't know about you, but I don't always have the time to sit down for a meal. And often I'm hungry with no healthy food in sight—all there is around me is a corner store near my next meeting or a coffee shop at my airport gate as I get ready for a flight.

So this hack is for those times—for real-life eating on the go, when we have to grab something on the way to the bus, when we're at a party or a business breakfast, rushing after work, or need to stop on the road. It's for those times when we're going to eat a slice of cake for breakfast because we're hungry and it's there.

The solution is simple, and I've mentioned it throughout these pages: combine starches and sugars with fat, protein, or fiber. So here's the hack: instead of letting carbs run around naked (on their own), put some "clothes" on them. Clothes on our carbs reduce how much and how quickly glucose is absorbed by our bodies.

Have the brownie at your friends' place, but ask for Greek yogurt with it, too. Have the bagel at the business meeting, but with some lox alongside. Buy a take-out lunch from a café, but add to it ingredients from a corner store salad bar: cherry tomatoes and some nuts. If you're making cookies, add nuts to the batter. If you're serving apple crumble, offer cream to go on top.

When you do enjoy carbs (and you will and should and must), make it a habit to add fiber, protein, or fat and, if you can, eat those first. Even savory snacks—which are already better for your glucose curves but may still contain starch—should have clothes on: add

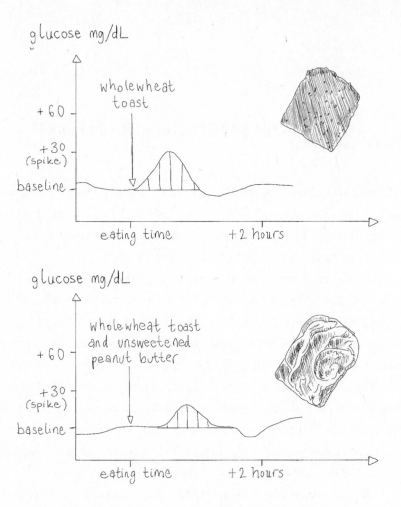

Often, putting clothes on your carbs makes them taste better, too.

avocado and cheese to toast, spread nut butter on rice cakes, and eat some almonds before your croissant.

I've heard that adding fat to a meal is bad because it increases the insulin spike.

This belief was popularized by a Frenchman, Michel Montignac, in the 1980s. But the most recent science demonstrates otherwise.

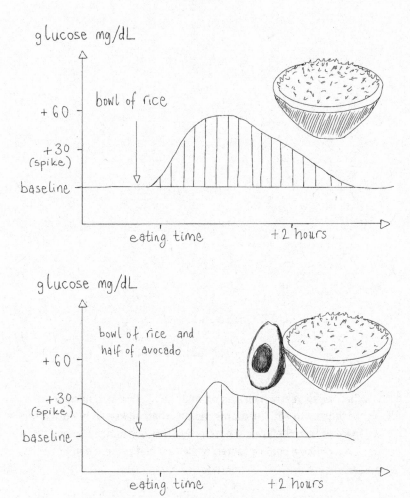

Rice is better for our glucose when it has clothes on.

Adding fat to a meal does not increase the insulin spike that meal causes. I repeat, adding fat to a meal does not increase the insulin spike. It does not tell our bodies to secrete more insulin. In fact, eating fat before a carb-rich meal *decreases* the amount of insulin produced in response to the meal.

Eating carbohydrates alone isn't just bad for our glucose levels, it also plays havoc with our hunger hormones. So we go from feeling full to being hungry again very quickly.

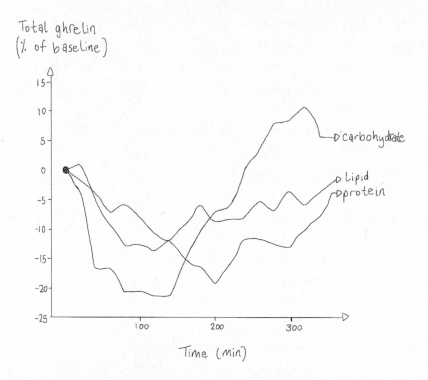

Total ghrelin
(% of baseline)

When we eat carbohydrates on their own, ghrelin, a hormone that tells us to eat, fluctuates rapidly, then makes us hungrier than we were before eating. Carbs drive our hunger up and down like a roller coaster, while fats and protein don't.

By putting clothes on our carbs, we avoid hunger pangs. We also avoid being *hangry*, something I experienced almost every day when I was a teenager.

MEET LUCY AND HER TEMPER

"I was concerned I would destroy all my relationships, one by one." This confession came out of the mouth of Lucy, 24, a heptathlon athlete who lives in the United Kingdom. Lucy was snapping at her parents and saying mean things to her friends. Her behavior was turning her into someone no one wanted to be around. As she came to dis-cover, she wasn't to blame—naked carbs were.

Thousands of scientific studies show how glucose spikes harm our body, but as I mentioned in the previous chapter, the fascinat-ing connection between glucose and the mind is still emerging. I've already described the research proving that the more glucose spikes in our diet, the more we feel symptoms of depression and anxiety. But thanks to a fascinating recent experiment, we also know that when we eat a breakfast that causes glucose spikes, we're more likely to want to punish those around us—we become vindictive and less agreeable to our peers.

Lucy's confession may seem extreme, but her glucose spikes were also extreme. This is because Lucy has type 1 diabetes. People with type 1 diabetes don't have the ability to make enough insulin. Without insulin, when a spike comes in, the glucose can't make its way into cells properly. So it stays very high in their bloodstream for very long, while the cells are starving for energy. This causes huge issues—before Lucy was diagnosed at 15 years old, she didn't even have enough energy to lift a fork.

On the first day of her new life as a type 1 diabetic, nurses at the hospital gave Lucy a plate of (naked) pasta to eat. They then taught her how to inject insulin with a syringe into her abdomen. The insulin diffused throughout her entire body, helping the glucose from the pasta make its way to the cells and bringing the spike caused by that pasta down.

The nurses explained: eat carbs at every meal and inject insulin at every meal. The bigger the glucose spike from what you just ate, the more insulin needs to be injected. This may sound simple to a nondiabetic, but getting the dosage right is a science. You have to constantly calculate where your glucose levels will be in the next hour or so, always planning ahead to avoid dreaded highs and lows. Eating, napping, exercising, all turn into a math problem. Huge spikes and huge drops are the name of the game for most people with type 1 diabetes. To give you an example, once diagnosed and using insulin, Lucy's glucose level would go up to 300 mg/dL, then down to 70 mg/dL, then back up to 250 mg/dL, and back down to 70 mg/dL on a daily basis. Remember, my biggest spike as a non-diabetic was from 100 mg/dL to 180 mg/dL from a doughnut on an empty stomach—and I felt the side effects keenly.

Lucy felt the side effects even more keenly. She woke up every morning feeling hungover. Whenever her glucose levels were high, she'd snap at her mother. She couldn't help it and regularly cried out of regret afterward. Home was one thing—until her teammates started avoiding her at school, too.

In me, a relatively small spike (compared to what someone with diabetes can experience) can trigger brain fog and depersonalization. In Lucy, spikes caused uncontrollable anger. She felt stuck, too. She thought, *I guess I have to live with this*.

Lucy started perusing the type 1 diabetic forums for advice on how to deal with her symptoms. Other people with type 1 diabetes were talking about flattening their glucose curves and linking to my Instagram account.

Lucy found a few things there that helped her: first, she saw that a nondiabetic, like myself, can also experience glucose spikes into the upper 180s. That was shocking to her. She had always thought that for nondiabetics, glucose levels remained stable between 80 and 100 mg/dL all day long. That made her feel less alone: it's hard for *all of us* to flatten our glucose curves.

Second, she saw I was wearing a glucose monitor. She said, "Seeing you wearing it proudly even though you don't need it gave me the courage to put one on too. It helped me not be embarrassed."

Finally, she saw that depending on what you eat, you really can flatten your glucose curves. Lucy understood that she could do something about how poorly she felt, body, mind, and soul.

She met with her endocrinologist and made a plan. (When you inject insulin or are on any type of medication, it's very important to talk to your doctor before changing the way you eat—to make sure you're not causing interactions that could be dangerous.)

Lucy had always been told to eat carbohydrates at every meal—and especially at breakfast. The first thing she did with her endocrinologist's supervision was to flatten her breakfast curve: from orange juice and croissants (which she didn't even like) to salmon, avocado, and almond milk. She used to see a spike of up to 300 mg/dL after breakfast. Now her glucose levels stay virtually flat.

Breakfast was easy to change, lunch and dinner as well, but snacks were less so. Lucy gets very hungry in the middle of the day because she trains so much, and she loves to reach for a banana or a candy bar.

What did she learn to do? To put some clothes on her carbs: she added nut butter to a banana, and she ate a hard-boiled egg before a candy bar. (A tip from Lucy: hard-boil eggs in batches every week, and keep them in your fridge.)

With these hacks, Lucy's HbA1c level (the measure of glucose variability) dropped from 7.4 to 5.1 in three months—5.1 is a level common among many nondiabetics. She injects about one-tenth the insulin she did before. And she's about ten times happier than before.

When we put clothes on our carbs, the game of Tetris our body plays with glucose goes from level 10 to level 1. There is less oxidative stress, fewer free radicals, less inflammation. And less insulin. With flatter glucose curves, we feel better and our mood is more stable.

Now, instead of feeling hungover, Lucy wakes up refreshed. It seems simple, but it's often the smallest things that are the most meaningful: She walks down to the kitchen with a smile on her face and asks her mother if she can make her a coffee. She doesn't get so angry anymore. She doesn't cry afterward if she snaps at

**If you're eating something sweet, put some clothes on it:
fiber, fat, or protein.**

her parents or her teammates—because she doesn't snap so often
these days.

   Her relationships are back to where she wants them. Her steady
glucose levels allow her, she said, to "be the person she wants to be,
just a nice person, and that's the most important."

   I've heard a lot of stories like these. Flatter curves can lead to our being more patient with our kids, more loving with our partner, and more supportive to our colleagues.

TRY THIS: Ever get hangry? Ever regret the way you speak to the people you love? Think about what you ate last before one of these situations occurred. You may be able to trace it back to naked carbs.

What about fruit?

As I explained in part 1, the fruit we eat these days has been bred for centuries to contain more glucose and fructose and less fiber than before. So although whole fruit is still the healthiest way to eat sugar, we can go a step further and help ourselves some more by combining it with glucose level–flattening friends—fat, protein, and fiber.

Turn the page for some tips to keep in mind.

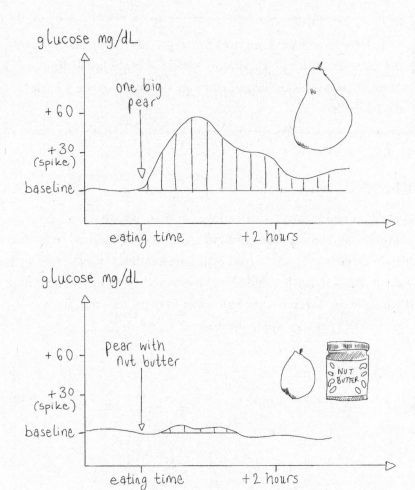

Combine your fruit—top favorite partners in the Glucose Goddess community are nut butter, nuts, full-fat yogurt, eggs, and cheddar cheese.

Dried dates are some of the biggest glucose bombs in the fruit
kingdom and spike us high even with clothes on them.
Yet they are said to help with managing diabetes. Go figure.
Really, it's best to avoid them or eat them in small quantities.

When you have a choice between various fruits, the best option is berries. Tropical fruits and grapes are bred to contain high amounts of sugar, so eat them for dessert or put some clothes on them.

Do whole grains still need clothes?

We often think that if grains are whole (brown rice, brown pasta, etc.), they are much better for us. The truth is, they are only very slightly better—starch is still starch. Pasta or bread that boasts "whole grain" on its package has still been milled—which means that some of its fiber is gone. If you want bread that contains beneficial fiber, choose a very dark bread, such as seed bread or pumpernickel (as mentioned in hack 2, "Add a green starter to all your meals").

In the end, rice is still rice, even if it's whole grain or wild rice. Don't let it go out naked. Mix in chopped fresh herbs, such as mint, parsley, and dill, and roasted nuts, such as almonds or pistachios, and enjoy it alongside roasted salmon or chicken. Voilà, your carbs are dressed to the nines—and to my mind, tastier, too.

Lentils and pulses are different, though: they are better for you than rice, because although rice (or pasta or bread) is 100 percent starch, lentils and pulses contain starch, fiber, *and* protein.

Remember: when we combine glucose with other molecules, whether we are diabetic or not, our body receives it at a more natural, manageable speed, and we curb the glucose spike.

If you're eating carbs on their own . . .

Bread, corn, couscous, pasta, polenta, rice, tortillas, cake, candy bars, cereal, cookies, crackers, fruit, granola, hot chocolate, ice cream, or anything else sweet

---

. . . combine them with fiber, fat, and/or protein:

Any vegetable, avocado, beans, butter, cheese, cream, eggs, fish, Greek yogurt, meat, nuts, seeds

---

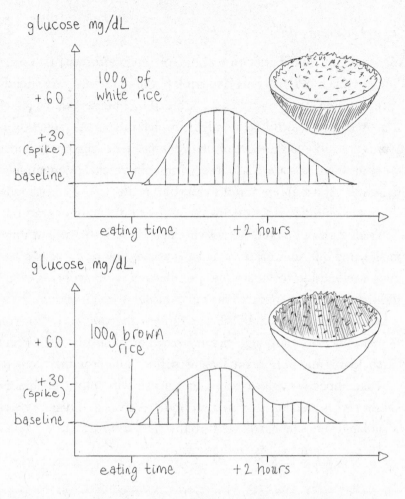

Brown rice is better than white rice for your glucose, but it's still rice. Try to give it some clothes to flatten its curve.

Which fat should I add?

Unlike sugar (there is no good or bad sugar; all sugar is the same, regardless of the plant it comes from), some fats are better for you than others.

Good fats are saturated (fat from animals, butter, ghee, and coconut oil) or monounsaturated (from fruit and nuts such as avocados, macadamia nuts, and olives). For cooking, use saturated fats—they're less likely to oxidize with heat. Monounsaturated fats, such as olive and avocado, can't stand the heat as well. A good rule of thumb to distinguish between them: cook with fats that are solid at room temperature when you can.

Bad fats (which inflame us, hurt our heart health, make us gain visceral fat, and increase our insulin resistance) are polyunsaturated and trans fats, which are found in processed oils—soybean oil, corn oil, canola oil, safflower oil, rice bran oil, fried foods, and fast foods. (The one seed oil that isn't as bad is flaxseed oil.)

We feel more satiated when there is fat in our diet, but we must be conscious of this dance: if we add *tons* of fat, our glucose spikes will be severely curbed, but we may start putting on weight. Add *some fat*, such as a tablespoon or two at a meal, but don't pour the entire bottle of olive oil onto your pasta.

Last, whenever you buy something, don't be fooled into thinking the "low-fat" version is better for you: 5% Greek yogurt will help your glucose curves much more than a low-fat yogurt will. (More on this in "How to spot a spike on a package" on page 209.)

How do I add fiber?

All veggies under the sun provide fiber. Along with nuts and seeds, they are the best clothes! You can even try fiber pills such as the ones made from psyllium husk.

How do I add protein?

Protein is found in animal products, such as eggs, meat, fish, dairy, and cheese, and also in many plant sources, such as nuts, seeds, and beans. You can also use protein powder. Look for those with only one ingredient listed: the source of the protein. I usually choose hemp, whey, or pea protein powder. Make sure there are no sweeteners in it.

I have type 1 diabetes. What should I do?

If you're going to change the way you eat in order to flatten your glucose curves, talk to your endocrinologist first. Adjusting your diet without adjusting your medication can cause unexpected highs and lows, and things could go wrong.

I have type 2 diabetes. What should I do?

If you're currently insulin dependent or taking any medication, speak to your doctor before making any changes to your diet. With proper support, many people can reverse their type 2 diabetes. Many Glucose Goddess community members have shared their stories of how with me. For instance, Laura, who is 57 years old, started her journey toward flattening her glucose curves at 300 pounds. She took metformin and glimepiride, two medications used to treat type 2 diabetes. After changing how she ate thanks to what she learned on my Instagram account and working closely with her doctor, she lost 50 pounds (and still counting), dropped her HbA1c level from 9 to 5.5, and reduced the dosage of her medications.

~~~~~

When I'm in Paris, where I live part of the time, I often go for a walk in the morning. At that time of day, when I pass a bakery, I really want to tear into a baguette. When we are hungry, naked carbs look very appealing. But I keep in mind that the hungrier I am, the emptier my stomach is, the bigger the spike those naked carbs will cause. (This is why flattening our breakfast curve is so important.) I developed the habit of dressing up that baguette: these days I'll snack on almonds from the corner store before my first bite of baguette, and when I get home, I'll spread some salted butter on it.

The hacks in this book have made a big difference in the lives of people in the Glucose Goddess community. I'm so excited for you to start trying them out, too. And as you do, remember: It's okay if you can't do them all the time. Even just adding them to your life a little bit, and when it's easy, will help your health.

CHEAT SHEETS
How to Be a Glucose Goddess
When Things Get Hard

Here are a few tips based on specific situations that people have asked me for advice about: when a craving hits, when we're at a bar, and when we're grocery shopping.

WHEN YOU'RE HAVING A CRAVING

Sometimes, even with all the hacks I've described in these pages, you may get hit with a craving for sugar. Here's how to beat it.

1. Give a craving a twenty-minute cooling-off period. Back in hunter-gatherer days, decreases in our glucose levels signaled that we hadn't eaten in a long time. In response, our brain told us to choose high-calorie foods. Today, when we encounter a decrease in glucose levels, it's usually because the last thing we ate caused a glucose spike. Yet our brain tells us to do the same thing, to choose high-calorie foods, even though we aren't famished—we've got energy

reserves. After a glucose drop, our liver quickly (within 20 minutes) steps in, releases stored glucose from those reserves into our bloodstream, and brings our levels back to normal. At that point, the craving often dissipates. So next time you're about to grab a cookie, set a timer for 20 minutes. If your craving was due to a glucose drop, it will be gone by the time the alarm rings.

2. If the 20 minutes have come and gone and you're still thinking about that cookie, set it aside for dessert at your next meal. In the meantime, consciously notice that you're having a craving and remind yourself that you've experienced this before and it will pass. Then try these craving killers: licorice root tea or a spoonful of coconut oil swirled into coffee. Other things to try: peppermint tea, pickle juice, gum, a big glass of water with a big pinch of salt. Brush your teeth. Or take a walk.

3. If you can't wait for dessert at your next meal and you've decided you're going to go ahead and eat what you're craving right now, drink a tall glass of water with a tablespoon of apple cider vinegar swirled in (or as close to a tablespoon as you like).

4. Then put some clothes on your carbs. Have an egg, a handful of nuts, a couple of spoonfuls of 5% Greek yogurt, or a head of roasted broccoli before the thing you're going to eat.

5. Eat that thing. Enjoy it!

6. Use your muscles and move within the next hour. Go for a walk or do some squats. Whatever works for you.

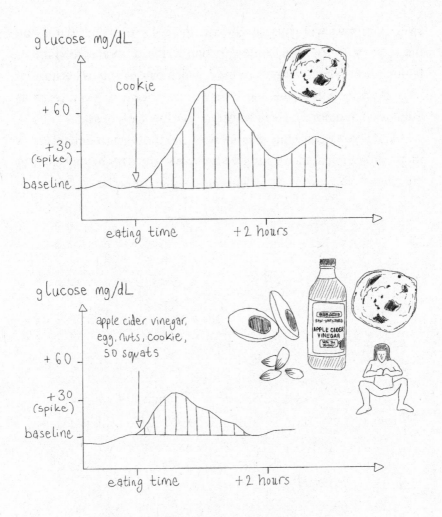

glucose mg/dL

cookie

+ 60

+ 30
(spike)

baseline

eating time   + 2 hours

glucose mg/dL

apple cider vinegar,
egg, nuts, cookie,
50 squats

+ 60

+ 30
(spike)

baseline

eating time   + 2 hours

Here is the ultimate hack combo to a craving.

WHEN YOU'RE AT A BAR

When you order a drink at a bar, you don't have to order a glucose and fructose spike along with it. (That is a lot for the liver to handle.)

Alcohols that keep our levels steady are wine (red, white, rosé, sparkling) as well as spirits (gin, vodka, tequila, whiskey, and even rum). We can drink these on an empty stomach, and they don't cause a glucose spike. Watch out for mixers: adding fruit juice, something sweet, or tonic will cause a glucose spike. Drink your alcohol on the rocks, with sparkling water or soda water, or with some lime or lemon juice. When it comes to beer, which causes spikes because of its high carb content, ale and lager are preferable to stout (such as Guinness) and porter. Even better, go for low-carb beer.

And if you're nibbling on appetizers, go for the nuts and olives, as those will help balance your glucose levels—and try to stay clear of the chips if you can, as those will cause a glucose spike.

If you're going to drink alcohol, wine is a better option than a cocktail.

WHEN YOU'RE GROCERY SHOPPING

You'll naturally flatten your glucose curves if you cut back on most processed foods, but for the occasions when you do buy processed foods, here's what to keep in mind.

The items on supermarket shelves don't get a gold star for honesty. Far from it. If a processed food will cause a glucose spike, it's not going to be up front about it on the package. It's going to hide that secret, distracting you with labels such as "fat free" or "no sugar added"—which unfortunately don't mean that the food is healthy. In order to find out if a processed food will cause a glucose spike, don't look at the front. Look at the back.

How to spot a spike on a package

The first place to look is the ingredients list. Ingredients are sorted in descending order by weight. If sugar is in the top five ingredients, that means a hefty proportion of that food consists of sugar—a soft white roll, for example, or ketchup—and will cause a glucose spike. If sugar is in the top five ingredients, the food will be sweet, and you know what that means: a hidden fructose spike.

Manufacturers have become very good at calling sugar by many names so that it's harder for consumers to figure out what's what. I know this is a little tedious, but I recommend reading through the list below at least once so that you see all the ingredients that will cause a spike.

The many names of sugar on an ingredients list

Look for these: agave nectar, agave syrup, barley malt, beet sugar, brown rice syrup, brown sugar, cane juice crystals, cane sugar, caramel, coconut sugar, confectioner's sugar, corn syrup, corn syrup solids, date sugar, crushed fruit, dextrin, dextrose, evaporated cane juice, fructose, fruit juice, fruit juice concentrate, fruit puree concentrate, galactose, glucose, glucose syrup solids, golden sugar, golden syrup, grape sugar, high-fructose corn syrup (HFCS), honey, icing sugar, malt syrup, maltodextrin, maltose, maple syrup, muscovado sugar, panela sugar, pressed fruit, raw sugar, rice syrup, sucanat, sucrose, sugar, turbinado sugar.

A special mention goes to "fruit juice," "fruit juice concentrate," "fruit puree concentrate," and "pressed fruit": more and more, these pop up on cereal boxes, yogurt containers, and granola boxes. As you now know, as soon as a fruit is denatured and processed and its fiber is extracted, it becomes sugar like any other sugar. When you pick up a juice or a smoothie, assess it as you would any other processed food: if the main ingredient is sugar—i.e., it is one of the "fruit" by-products listed above—skip it. Eat a peach or apple instead.

The ingredients list on an Innocent smoothie: sugar under four different names (and a dash of lemon juice). I know they look cute, but remember, fruit juice is just sugar.

German candy made with
25 percent fruit juice.

INGREDIENTS: WHEAT FLOUR, SUGAR, VEGETABLE GLYCERIN, FRUCTOSE, DEXTROSE, MALTODEXTRIN, VEGETABLE AND MODIFIED PALM OIL SHORTENING, PALM KERNEL AND/OR PALM OIL, MODIFIED CORN STARCH, APPLE POWDER, PALM OIL, MODIFIED MILK INGREDIENTS, STRAWBERRY PUREE CONCENTRATE, CORN STARCH, BAKING POWDER, SOY LECITHIN, SALT, ACETYLATED TARTARIC ACID ESTERS OF MONO- AND DIGLYCERIDES, COLOUR (CARROT JUICE CONCENTRATE), SODIUM CITRATE, NATURAL FLAVOUR, CELLULOSE GEL, CITRIC ACID, MALIC ACID, MONO- AND DIGLYCERIDES, CELLULOSE GUM, SODIUM ALGINATE.
CONTAINS WHEAT, MILK AND SOY INGREDIENTS.

The ingredients in Special K fruit crisp bars. Can you find the six different sugar names listed here?

Stick to the facts

Sometimes it seems as though every single part of packaging is trying to confuse us. But I'm happy to announce that there is one haven of objective information: the Nutrition Facts.

One thing to keep in mind before we begin: in recent years manufacturers have been reducing the recommended serving sizes on their packages to make things look better in terms of grams of sugar. A smaller serving size means less sugar per serving. But come on, who eats only *two* Oreos? So know that the absolute numbers you see on packaging are not the most important thing. Rather, it's the *ratios* that hold the key. Let me explain this powerful way to decode things.

First things first: you can skip right past the Calories line. Yes, it's the line in the biggest type, because that's what manufacturers want you to focus on. But as I've explained, the molecules matter more than the calories. And in the Nutrition Facts, the molecules in a food are spelled out for all to see—if you know where to look.

When assessing dry foods, such as cookies, pasta, bread, cereal, cereal bars, crackers, and chips, head to the Total Carbohydrate section. The grams next to Total Carbohydrate and Total Sugars represent the molecules that cause a glucose spike: starches and sugars. The more grams of these, the more the food will lead to a rise in your

.

Nutrition Facts

Serving size

Amount Per Serving

Calories 0

	% Daily Value*
Total Fat 0g	0%
Saturated Fat 0g	0%
Trans Fat 0g	
Sodium 0mg	0%
Total Carbohydrate 0g	0%
Dietary Fiber 0g	0%
Total Sugars 0g	
Includes 0g Added Sugars	0%
Protein 0g	0%

Not a significant source of cholesterol, vitamin D, calcium, iron, and potassium

*The % Daily Value (DV) tells you how much a nutrient in a serving of food contributes to a daily diet. 2,000 calories a day is used for general nutrition advice.

On a Nutrition Facts label on packaged food, calories may be what's written in the biggest type, but it's not what will tell you whether the food is going to cause a spike or not.

glucose, fructose, and insulin levels and set off the chain reaction that keeps you craving sweet things.

This section also contains the Dietary Fiber line, and as I've described throughout this book, fiber is the only carbohydrate that our bodies don't break down—the more fiber in the food, the flatter the glucose curve after eating it. So here's a tip: for dry foods, look at the ratio of Total Carbohydrate to Dietary Fiber.

Select items whose ingredients get the closest to 1 gram of Dietary Fiber for each 5 grams of Total Carbohydrate. Here's how to do it: find the number next to Total Carbohydrate and divide it by five. Try to find a food that has that amount of Dietary Fiber (or as close to it as possible).

Why five? It's an arbitrary cutoff, but I use it because it's close to the ratio we find in fruit such as berries. The science is not exact, but I have found that the closer the food is to this ratio, the flatter the curve it will cause.

Let's say you need to buy bread. Go to the grocery store with

Nutrition Facts		
15 servings per container		
Serving size		**30g**

Amount per serving		
Calories		**60**

	% Daily Value*
Total Fat 1g	1%
Saturated Fat 0g	0%
Trans Fat 0g	
Cholesterol 0mg	0%
Sodium 110mg	4%
Total Carbohydrate 25g	8%
Dietary Fiber 14g	57%
Total Sugars 0g	
Includes 0g Added Sugars	0%
Protein 2g	
Vitamin D 2mcg	10%
Calcium 260mg	20%
Iron 8mg	45%
Potassium 240mg	6%

* The % Daily Value (DV) tells you how much a nutrient in a serving of food contributes to a daily diet. 2,000 calories a day is used for general nutrition advice.

Nutrition Facts		
15 servings per container		
Serving size		**29g**

Amount per serving		
Calories		**100**

	% Daily Value*
Total Fat 0g	0%
Saturated Fat 0g	0%
Trans Fat 0g	
Cholesterol 0mg	0%
Sodium 190mg	8%
Total Carbohydrate 25g	8%
Dietary Fiber 2g	8%
Total Sugars 7g	
Includes 7g Added Sugars	
Protein 2g	
Vitamin D	20%
Calcium	
Iron	30%
Potassium	2%

* The % Daily Value (DV) tells you how much a nutrient in a serving of food contributes to a daily diet. 2,000 calories a day is used for general nutrition advice.

Compare these two cereal labels: Fiber One on the left, Special K on the right. The one on the left has a better fiber-to-carb ratio (14 grams of fiber per 25 grams of total carbs versus 2 grams of fiber per 25 grams of total carbs). The one on the left is a better choice.

your shopping list. Compare options to find items that will keep your spikes low. Put down any loaves that list sugar in their top five ingredients, and of the others choose the one that has the most Dietary Fiber per gram of Total Carbohydrate. Voilà!

TRY THIS: Grab something in your pantry that you eat often. Turn to the back of the box and check whether it will cause a spike. Is sugar in the top five ingredients? Is there at least 1 gram of fiber for each 5 grams of total carbohydrate?

Can I combine these foods with protein and fiber from a different source?

Yes, absolutely you can. You can always buy a food that could cause a spike, and then, when you eat it, combine it with fiber, protein, and fat—like Oreos with Greek yogurt and nuts. But you'll make it easier on yourself if you start with ingredients that will help keep your glucose levels steady anyway.

Should I never buy anything that spikes me or that has sugar in the top three ingredients?

No, no, that would be draconian! The most important thing is to be aware of what spikes you and what doesn't. When I buy ice cream, I'm buying a food that has a ton of sugar in it. It will definitely cause a glucose spike. I know that. It's a conscious decision. I eat it on occasion, rather than every day. For things such as yogurt and bread, which I do eat every day, I buy the versions I know will keep my glucose levels steady.

BEWARE OF THE LIES

Here is some of the most fun detective work to do—just because a package says something cool on the front doesn't mean that it is good for you. The following fancy marketing claims and packaging are just trying to get you to buy their products. For instance, gluten-free, vegan, and organic do not mean that the food won't spike you.

"Gluten free" doesn't mean "healthy." It just means the food wasn't made with wheat. It can still contain other starches and loads of sugar.

"Vegan" doesn't mean "healthy." It just means the food contains no animal products. Same as gluten-free things, these can contain a bunch of starch and sugar.

**"Organic" doesn't mean "healthy." The food
can still contain loads of starch and sugar.**

TRY THIS: At the grocery store, stay in the outside aisles. If you shop on the outskirts, you'll find fruit, veggies, dairy, meat, fish— all minimally processed foods. If you venture into the middle aisles, make sure to use the techniques in this chapter to choose processed foods well. Pretty soon, your brain will become a spike-scanning machine.

And one last tip: Never go shopping hungry . . . it messes with your brain. When I do, all vegetables look highly unappetizing, and every chocolatey item on the shelves calls my name.

A Day in the Life of a Glucose Goddess

U sing the hacks in this book, there are many ways to live like a Glucose God or Goddess. Here is an example from my own life, where I use the hacks in this book to flatten my glucose curves.

Breakfast: I had coffee with a splash of whole, not skim, milk; the higher fat content helped keep my glucose steady. Two eggs scrambled in a pan with butter and sea salt, served with a couple tablespoons of hummus on the side. Then a slice of toasted dark rye bread with butter. Before going out the door, I grabbed a square of 80 percent dark chocolate—I wanted something sweet, and it's best to eat it at the end of a meal rather than on its own at 11 a.m., as I used to do.

Hacks I used:

- Hack 4: Flatten your breakfast curve.
- Hack 6: Pick dessert over a sweet snack.

At work: I had black tea (I usually have green tea, but we were out of it).

Lunch: I microwaved leftovers from the night before: green beans, tahini-baked cod, and wild rice, which I ate in that exact order.

The hack I used:

- Hack 1: Eat foods in the right order.

Afternoon: While on a walk, I came across the best-looking cookie in the world. So I pulled out a tool from my toolbox: I bought the cookie but didn't eat it just then. I got back to the office, drank a glass of water with a tablespoon of apple cider vinegar swirled in, then five almonds, *then* ate the cookie. About 20 minutes later, it was time to use my muscles to help flatten the curve. So I headed to the bathroom, and there I did 30 squats and 10 push-ups against the sink.
Hacks I used:

- Hack 7: Reach for vinegar before you eat.
- Hack 10: Put some clothes on your carbs.
- Hack 8: After you eat, move.

Dinner: I had friends over for dinner. I served crudités—raw carrots and sliced hearts of palm—as an appetizer. Once we sat down, I brought out my favorite ham salad and rosemary oven-roasted potatoes on the side. My friends know by now to eat the salad first, then the potatoes, to flatten their glucose curves.

Dessert was strawberries and clotted cream. Twenty minutes after finishing dessert, I got everybody up and we went for a 10-minute walk outside to the local square. When we got back, my guests were so energized that they all wanted to help with the dishes!
Hacks I used:

- Hack 1: Eat foods in the right order.
- Hack 2: Add a green starter to all your meals.
- Hack 10: Put some clothes on your carbs.
- Hack 8: After you eat, move.

You Are Special

The hacks in this book will work for all of us. No matter who you are, eating your carbs last and adding a green starter to your meal will always flatten your glucose curve. A savory breakfast is the way to go. Vinegar and exercise will enable you to eat your cake and have health, too.

However, within a specific category of food—say, dessert—the best option for one person may differ from the best option for her neighbor.

In 2019 I helped my friend Luna get fitted with a glucose monitor and recruited her for a very challenging experiment. First, we ate the exact same breakfast and lunch that didn't spike us. Then, in the middle of the afternoon, I baked cookies, took ice cream out of the freezer, and asked her to eat them at the same time as I did.

What happened was mind-blowing.

A humongous spike for me, barely a spike for her. Neither of us exercised for two hours before or two hours after eating, and no vinegar was consumed. You may be wondering what the heck is going on. Why did the cookies and ice cream shoot my glucose levels through the roof but not hers?

This wasn't a fluke or an isolated experiment. Starting in 2015, research teams around the world have found the same peculiar

Two people can have different glucose responses to the same food.

result: the same food can create different responses depending on the person.

These differences are due to many factors: the amount of baseline insulin we have, our muscle mass, different gut microbes, being more or less hydrated, being more or less rested, being more or less stressed, whether or not we have just worked out (or we work out after eating)—the list goes on. Some studies even found that if you *think* you're about to eat something sugary, that can cause the food to cause a bigger spike for you than someone else.

But although the peaks of our respective spikes may have been different, the general principle applies: if Luna and I had eaten nuts before our cookies and ice cream, both our spikes would have been proportionally smaller.

Individual differences become useful when we look at categories of food. For example, if we look at cookies, that particular food wasn't a good choice for me, while it was probably fine for Luna. So if I'm craving something sweet, I know that cookies aren't the best option for me, whereas apple pie I can handle quite well.

Again, this is rather incomplete. Luna might have had a small spike because she had more insulin in her body—in which case this could actually point to her being less metabolically healthy than me. Science still has a way to go here.

The hacks in this book work for everyone—you don't need to wear a continuous glucose monitor to use them. But if you someday wear a continuous glucose monitor, you may find specific foods that work well for you.

To go even further, you may combine the data from a continuous glucose monitor with an analysis of your gut microbiome, and with your blood fat response to foods. Tim Spector, who provided a blurb for this book, is a scientist who started a company named Zoe that does just that. I've tested the product—it's clear to me that it's what the future is made of.

The End

I am humbled and lucky to hear from many of you every day, and in your messages there is one resounding conclusion: Regardless of what your diet is, your lifestyle, your age, where you live, your past struggles with health, applying the hacks has made a big difference in your lives. As I finish this book and write these words at home in Paris, I want to thank you for giving me the opportunity to share this science.

I know how hard it can be, trying to keep yourself well. Many of us have felt misguided, with conflicting messages coming from all corners. For a long time, I did, too. Indeed, there are many problems with the food advice we get these days, not the least of which is that it is rarely totally impartial.

Maybe because of this you've been following one health regime or another that has not only not worked but has made your condition worse. Maybe your body has felt like a black box. Maybe you've felt tired for years; maybe you're battling cravings or weight gain or a chronic condition. Maybe you are depressed, have fertility troubles, or are inching closer and closer to type 2 diabetes. Maybe you're lost as to how to manage your type 1 diabetes or your gestational diabetes. Maybe you take medication for a condition you were told you can't do anything about.

I hope you have learned from reading this book that the symptoms you are having are actually powerful messages. Your body is speaking to you.

My aim has been to bring up-to-date, objective science into the realm of action, to turn unbiased research into realistic tools, to arm you with knowledge about how your body works, and to help you feel amazing.

What are you going to do? Are you going to listen to your body, understand the glucose lever in the cockpit, and get yourself back to cruising altitude? I hope you are. As you do, remember, it's important to be kind to yourself in the process. I hope you will then go on to help your parents, siblings, children, friends, and acquaintances do the same. Together we can help everyone reconnect with their bodies, one person at a time. I hope you'll let me know how it goes. I'd love to hear about your journey. Reach out to me on Instagram at @glucosegoddess.

Acknowledgments

This book took a village. And what a village! I'd like to thank the people in the Glucose Goddess community who contributed their glucose data, their stories, and their passion to this work. This book was born out of the movement that we're building together.

I'd like to thank Susanna Lea, agent of my dreams, for bringing her experience, humor, and wisdom to my life. Thank you to Mark Kessler and everyone at SLA for welcoming me. Thank you to the team at Simon & Schuster and to Emily Graff for your enthusiasm and commitment. Thank you to Short Books, to Rebecca Nicolson and Aurea Carpenter for your force and dedication. Thank you, Evie Dunne, for your brilliant illustrations.

Thank you to Robert Lustig for the feedback that I terribly needed. Thank you to Elissa Burnside, my first friend and my first reader, for your spirit and love. Thank you to Franklin Servan-Schreiber for channeling the universe for me. Thank you to David Servan-Schreiber for paving the way.

To my friends, thank you for being the best and for sharing this adventure with me. Dario, thank you for embodying the word *gift*. Thank you, Sefora, for helping me through my life. Thank you to Alice, Paul, Ines, Mathieu, Arthur, Jasmyn, and my entire family.

Thank you, Dad, for your kindness. Thank you, Mom, for being *my* goddess.

Thank you to Anne Wojcicki, Kevin Ryan, and Thomas Sherman for believing in me and guiding my path.

Thank you to all the scientists who ran the studies around the world, and to those before them, whose shoulders this work rests upon. Thank you to Axel Esselmann and Lauren Kohatsu for believing in this work from the beginning. Thank you to everyone at 23andMe who shaped my understanding of how we can make science accessible. Thank you, Bo, for your help getting this crazy project off the ground.

Closing this book out, I also want to say thank you to myself. Thank you for trusting and following what makes your soul light up. Waking up and going after it. While it wasn't an easy journey, I'm glad the idea picked me—and I hope I did it justice.

HOW I GOT HERE

xxv *Your genes can increase your likelihood of developing type 2 diabetes*: Michael Multhaup et al., *The Science Behind 23andMe's Type 2 Diabetes Report*, 2019, accessed August 30, 2021, https://permalinks.23andme.com/pdf/23_19-Type2Diabetes_March2019.pdf.

xxvi *Top athletes started to wear CGMs, too*: Mark Hearris et al., "Regulation of muscle glycogen metabolism during exercise: implications for endurance performance and training adaptations," *Nutrients* 10, no. 3 (2018): 298.

xxvi *Nondiabetics could have highly dysregulated glucose levels*: Heather Hall et al., "Glucotypes reveal new patterns of glucose dysregulation," *PLoS Biology* 16, no. 7 (2018): e2005143, https://pubmed.ncbi.nlm.nih.gov/30040822/.

1: ENTER THE COCKPIT

4 *Only 12 percent of Americans are metabolically healthy*: Joana Araújo et al., "Prevalence of Optimal Metabolic Health in American Adults: National Health and Nutrition Examination Survey 2009–2016," *Metabolic Syndrome and Related Disorders* 17, no. 1 (2019): 46–52, https://pubmed.ncbi.nlm.nih.gov/30484738/.

4 *Waist size is better for predicting underlying disease than BMI is*: Division of Nutrition, Physical Activity, and Obesity, National Center for Chronic Disease Prevention and Health Promotion, *Assessing Your Weight*, CDC, September 17, 2020, accessed August 30, 2021, https://www.cdc.gov/healthyweight/assessing/index.html.

2: MEET JERRY

12 *Plants make extra glucose during the day*: Gregory MacNeill et al., "Starch as a source, starch as a sink: the bifunctional role of starch in carbon allocation," *Journal of Experimental Botany* 68, no. 16 (2017): 4433–53, https://pubmed.ncbi.nlm.nih.gov/28981786/.

15 *Plants also transform some of their glucose into an* extra-sweet *molecule called* fructose: M. D. Joesten et al., "Sweetness relative to sucrose (table)," in *The World of Chemistry: Essentials*, 4th ed. (Pacific Grove, CA: Thomson Brooks/Cole, 2007), 359.

Notes

DEAR READER

xvi   *What we eat affects the 30 trillion cells*: Ron Sender et al., "Revised estimates for the number of human and bacteria cells in the body," *PLoS Biology* 14, no. 8 (2016): e1002533.

xvi   *Our nutritional choices are influenced by billion-dollar marketing campaigns*: Rudd Center for Food Policy and Obesity, *Increasing Disparities in Unhealthy Food Advertising Targeted to Hispanic and Black Youth*, January 2019, accessed August 30, 2021, https://media.rudd center.uconn.edu/PDFs/TargetedMarketingReport2019.pdf.

xvi   *These are usually justified under*: Robert H. Lustig, *Metabolical: The Lure and the Lies of Processed Food, Nutrition, and Modern Medicine* (New York: Harper Wave, 2021).

xvi   *Processed foods and sugar are inherently bad*: Lustig, *Metabolical*.

xviii   *88 percent of Americans are likely to have dysregulated glucose levels*: Joana Araújo et al., "Prevalence of Optimal Metabolic Health in American Adults: National Health and Nutrition Examination Survey 2009–2016," *Metabolic Syndrome and Related Disorders* 17, no. 1 (2019): 46–52.

xviii   *Too much insulin is one of the main drivers of*: Benjamin Bikman, *Why We Get Sick: The Hidden Epidemic at the Root of Most Chronic Diseases and How to Fight It* (New York: BenBella, 2020).

xix   *Too much fructose increases the likelihood of*: Lustig, *Metabolical*.

3: A FAMILY AFFAIR

17 *Every* second, *your body burns*: The body uses 200 grams of glucose daily. Glucose has a molar mass of 180 g/mole. Per day, the body therefore uses 0.1111 mole of glucose. One mole has 6.02214076×1023 molecules in it. So the body uses 6.6912675e+23 molecules of glucose per day. A day has 86,400 seconds in it: 7.7445226e+18 molecules per second. Jeremy M. Berg, *Biochemistry,* 5th ed. (New York: W. H. Freeman, 2002), Section 30.2.

17 *If each glucose molecule were a grain of sand*: About 5 sextillion (5 x 10"21 grains of sand on earth). Jason Marshall, *How Many Grains of Sand Are on Earth's Beaches?* Quick and Dirty Tips, 2016, accessed August 30, 2021, https://www.quickanddirtytips.com/education/math/how-many-grains-of-sand-are-on-earth-s-beaches?page=all.

18 *Using the same enzyme that plants use*: Liangliang Ju et al., "New insights into the origin and evolution of a-amylase genes in green plants," *Scientific Reports* 9, no. 1 (2019): 1–12, https://pubmed.ncbi.nlm.nih.gov/30894656/.

19 *Fructose is a little more complicated*: Cholsoon Jang et al., "The small intestine converts dietary fructose into glucose and organic acids," *Cell Metabolism* 27, no. 2 (2018): 351–61, https://www.ncbi.nlm.nih.gov/pmc/articles/PMC6032988/#SD1.

21 *In 1969, a cohort of scientists wrote a*: IUPAC, Comm, and IUPAC–IUB Comm, "Tentative rules for carbohydrate nomenclature. Part 1, 1969," *Biochemistry* 10, no. 21 (1971): 3983–4004, https://pubs.acs.org/doi/abs/10.1021/bi00797a028.

22 *Some humans evolved in areas without*: Mindy Weisberger, "Unknown Group of Ancient Humans Once Lived in Siberia, New Evidence Reveals," *Live Science*, 2019, accessed August 30, 2021, https://www.livescience.com/65654-dna-ice-age-teeth-siberia.html.

23 *Scientists know that humans' prehistoric diet*: Marion Nestle, "Paleolithic diets: A Sceptical View," *Nutrition Bulletin* 25.1 (2000): 43–47, https://onlinelibrary.wiley.com/doi/abs/10.1046/j.1467-3010.2000.00019.x.

23 *They adapted to the unique food supply*: Peter Ungar, *Evolution's Bite: A Story of Teeth, Diet, and Human Origins* (Princeton, NJ: Princeton University Press, 2017).

4: SEEKING PLEASURE

26   *Fiber-packed seeds*: U.S. Department of Agriculture, "Wheat bran, crude," FoodData Central, 2019, accessed August 30, 2019, https://fdc.nal.usda.gov/fdc-app.html#/food-details/169722/nutrients.

26   *Starchy bread*: U.S. Department of Agriculture, "Bread, white, commercially prepared," FoodData Central, 2019, accessed August 30, 2019, https://fdc.nal.usda.gov/fdc-app.html#/food-details/325871/nutrients.

27   *This is the same chemical that is released*: Nora Volkow et al., "The brain on drugs: from reward to addiction," *Cell* no. 162.4 (2015): 712–25, https://pubmed.ncbi.nlm.nih.gov/26276628/.

27   *In a 2016 study, mice were given a lever*: Vincent Pascoli et al., "Sufficiency of mesolimbic dopamine neuron stimulation for the progression to addiction," *Neuron* 88, no. 5 (2015): 1054–66, http://www.addictionscience.unige.ch/files/8214/6037/1136/NeuronVP2015.pdf.

28   *Ancestral bananas*: Australia & Pacific Science Foundation, "Tracing antiquity of banana cultivation in Papua New Guinea," AP Science, http://www.apscience.org.au/pbf_02_3/.

28   *On the left, a peach as it was*: Genetic Literacy Project, "How your food would look if not genetically modified over millennia," GLP, 2014, https://geneticliteracyproject.org/2014/06/19/how-your-food-would-look-if-not-genetically-modified-over-millennia/.

29   *Fruit, such as cherries*: U.S. Department of Agriculture, "Cherries, sweet, raw," FoodData Central, 2019, accessed August 30, 2019, https://fdc.nal.usda.gov/fdc-app.html#/food-details/171719/nutrients.

29   *Candy, such as jelly beans*: U.S. Department of Agriculture, "Candies, jellybeans," FoodData Central, 2019, accessed August 30, 2019, https://fdc.nal.usda.gov/fdc-app.html#/food-details/167991/nutrients.

29   *Sugar has become ever more concentrated*: Robert H. Lustig, *Metabolical: The Lure and the Lies of Processed Food, Nutrition, and Modern Medicine* (New York: Harper Wave, 2021).

29   *It's hard for our brain to curb its cravings*: Kevin Hall et al., "Ultra-processed diets cause excess calorie intake and weight gain: an inpatient randomized controlled trial of ad libitum food intake," *Cell Metabolism* 30, no. 1 (2019): 67–77, https://www.cell.com/action/showPdf?pii=S1550-4131(19)30248-7.

29   *Even tomatoes have been turned*: U.S. Department of Agriculture, "Tomato, roma," FoodData Central, 2021, accessed August 30, 2019, https://fdc.nal.usda.gov/fdc-app.html#/food-details/1750354/nutrients.

29   *Ketchup*: U.S. Department of Agriculture, "Ketchup, restaurant,"
     FoodData Central, 2019, accessed August 30, 2019, https://fdc.nal.usda
     .gov/fdc-app.html#/food-details/747693/nutrients.

30   *It gives us pleasure*: Robert H. Lustig, *The Hacking of the American
     Mind: The Science Behind the Corporate Takeover of Our Bodies and
     Brains* (New York: Penguin, 2017).

5: UNDERNEATH OUR SKIN

32   *The American Diabetes Association (ADA) states that*: American Di-
     abetes Association, "Understanding A1C: Diagnosis," *Diabetes*, ac-
     cessed August 30, 2019, https://www.diabetes.org/a1c/diagnosis.

32   *More likelihood of developing health problems from 85 mg/dL*: Jørgen
     Bjørnholt et al., "Fasting blood glucose: an underestimated risk factor
     for cardiovascular death. Results from a 22-year follow-up of healthy
     nondiabetic men," *Diabetes Care* 22, no. 1 (1999): 45–49, https://care
     .diabetesjournals.org/content/22/1/45.

32   *More likelihood of developing health problems from 85 mg/dL*: Chan-
     shin Park et al., "Fasting glucose level and the risk of incident ath-
     erosclerotic cardiovascular diseases," *Diabetes Care* 36, no. 7 (2013):
     1988–93, https://care.diabetesjournals.org/content/36/7/1988.

32   *More likelihood of developing health problems from 85 mg/dL*: Quoc
     Manh Nguyen et al., "Fasting plasma glucose levels within the normo-
     glycemic range in childhood as a predictor of prediabetes and type 2 di-
     abetes in adulthood: the Bogalusa Heart Study," *Archives of Pediatrics
     & Adolescent Medicine* 164, no. 2 (2010): 124–28, https://jamanetwork
     .com/journals/jamapediatrics/fullarticle/382778.

33   *Studies in nondiabetics give more precise information*: Guido Freck-
     mann et al., "Continuous glucose profiles in healthy subjects under
     everyday life conditions and after different meals," *Journal of Diabetes
     Science and Technology* 1, no. 5 (2007): 695–703, https://www.ncbi.nlm
     .nih.gov/pmc/articles/PMC2769652/.

33   *It's the* variability *caused by spikes that is most problematic*: Antonio
     Ceriello et al., "Oscillating glucose is more deleterious to endothelial
     function and oxidative stress than mean glucose in normal and type 2
     diabetic patients," *Diabetes* 57, no. 5 (2008): 1349–54, https://diabetes
     .diabetesjournals.org/content/57/5/1349.short.

33   *It's the* variability *caused by spikes that is most problematic*: Louis Mon-
     nier et al., "Activation of oxidative stress by acute glucose fluctuations

compared with sustained chronic hyperglycemia in patients with type 2 diabetes," *JAMA* 295, no. 14 (2006): 1681–87, https://jamanetwork.com /journals/jama/article-abstract/202670.

33   *It's the* variability *caused by spikes that is most problematic*: Giada Acciaroli et al., "Diabetes and prediabetes classification using glycemic variability indices from continuous glucose monitoring data," *Journal of Diabetes Science and Technology* 12, no. 1 (2018): 105–113, https:// www.ncbi.nlm.nih.gov/pmc/articles/PMC5761967/.

34   *The smaller your glycemic variability*: Zheng Zhou et al., "Glycemic variability: adverse clinical outcomes and how to improve it?" *Cardiovascular Diabetology* 19, no. 1 (2020): 1–14, https://link.springer.com /article/10.1186/s12933-020-01085-6.

6: TRAINS, TOAST, AND TETRIS

41   *More than 30 trillion cells*: Ron Sender et al., "Revised estimates for the number of human and bacteria cells in the body," *PLoS Biology* 14, no. 8 (2016): e1002533, https://journals.plos.org/plosbiology/article ?id=10.1371/journal.pbio.1002533.

43   *The Allostatic Load Model*: Martin Picard et al., "Mitochondrial allostatic load puts the 'gluc' back in glucocorticoids," *Nature Reviews Endocrinology* 10, no. 5 (2014): 303–10, https://www.uclahealth.org /reversibility-network/workfiles/resources/publications/picard-endo crinol.pdf.

43   *Free radicals*: Biplab Giri et al., "Chronic hyperglycemia mediated physiological alteration and metabolic distortion leads to organ dysfunction, infection, cancer progression and other pathophysiological consequences: an update on glucose toxicity," *Biomedicine & Pharmacotherapy*, no. 107 (2018): 306–28, https://www.sciencedirect.com /science/article/pii/S0753332218322406#fig0005.

44   *Oxidative stress is a driver of*: Picard, "Mitochondrial allostatic load," 303–10.

44   *Fructose increases oxidative stress even more*: Robert H. Lustig, "Fructose: it's 'alcohol without the buzz,'" *Advances in Nutrition* 4, no. 2 (2013): 226–35, https://www.ncbi.nlm.nih.gov/pmc/articles/PM C3649103/.

44   *Too much fat can also increase oxidative stress*: Joseph Evans et al., "Are oxidative stress-activated signaling pathways mediators of insu-

lin resistance and ß-cell dysfunction?" *Diabetes* 52, no. 1 (2003): 1–8, https://diabetes.diabetesjournals.org/content/52/1/1.short.

45 *You are* browning, *just like a slice of bread*: Jaime Uribarri et al., "Advanced glycation end products in foods and a practical guide to their reduction in the diet," *Journal of the American Dietetic Association* 100, no. 6 (2010): 911–16, https://www.ncbi.nlm.nih.gov/pmc/articles/PMC3704564/.

45 *When scientists look at the rib cage cartilage*: D. G. Dyer et al., "The Maillard reaction in vivo," *Zeitschrift für Ernährungswissenschaft* 30, no. 1 (1991): 29–45, https://www.researchgate.net/publication/21298 410_The_Maillard_reaction_in_vivo.

45 *This process is a normal and inevitable part of life*: Chan-Sik Kim et al., "The role of glycation in the pathogenesis of aging and its prevention through herbal products and physical exercise," *Journal of Exercise, Nutrition & Biochemistry* 21, no. 3 (2017): 55, https://www.ncbi .nlm.nih.gov/pmc/articles/PMC5643203.

46 *Consequences of glycated molecules range from wrinkles*: Masamitsu Ichihashi et al., "Glycation stress and photo-aging in skin," *Anti-Aging Medicine* 8, no. 3 (2011): 23–29, https://www.jstage.jst.go.jp/arti cle/jaam/8/3/8_3_23/_article/-char/ja/.

46 *Cataracts*: Ashok Katta et al., "Glycation of lens crystalline protein in the pathogenesis of various forms of cataract," *Biomedical Research* 20, no. 2 (2009): 119–21, https://www.researchgate.net/profile /Ashok-Katta-3/publication/233419577_Glycation_of_lens_crystalline _protein_in_the_pathogenesis_of_various_forms_of_cataract/links /02e7e531342066c955000000/Glycation-of-lens-crystalline-protein -in-the-pathogenesis-of-various-forms-of-cataract.pdf.

46 *Heart disease*: Georgia Soldatos et al., "Advanced glycation end products and vascular structure and function," *Current Hypertension Reports* 8, no. 6 (2006): 472–78, https://pubmed.ncbi.nlm.nih.gov/17087858/.

46 *Alzheimer's disease*: Masayoshi Takeuchi et al., "Involvement of advanced glycation end-products (AGEs) in Alzheimer's disease," *Current Alzheimer Research* 1, no. 1 (2004): 39–46, https://www.ingenta connect.com/content/ben/car/2004/00000001/00000001/art00006.

46 *Slowing down the browning reaction in your body leads to a longer life*: Kim, "The role of glycation in the pathogenesis of aging," 55.

46 *Fructose molecules glycate things* 10 times: Alejandro Gugliucci, "Formation of fructose-mediated advanced glycation end products and their roles in metabolic and inflammatory diseases," *Advances in*

*Nutrition*8,no.1(2017):54–62,https://www.ncbi.nlm.nih.gov/pmc/articles/PMC5227984/.

46   *Inflammation-based diseases "the greatest threat to human health"*: Roma Pahwa et al., "Chronic Inflammation," (2018), https://www.ncbi.nlm.nih.gov/books/NBK493173/.

46   *Three out of five people will die of an inflammation-based disease*: Pahwa, "Chronic inflammation."

48   *Glycogen is actually the cousin of starch*: Jeremy M. Berg, *Biochemistry*, 5th ed. (New York: W. H. Freeman and Co., 2002).

48   *The liver can hold about 100 grams of glucose*: David H. Wasserman, "Four grams of glucose," *American Journal of Physiology-Endocrinology and Metabolism* 296, no. 1 (2009): E11–E21, https://www.ncbi.nlm.nih.gov/pmc/articles/PMC2636990/.

48   *That's half of the 200 grams*: Berg, *Biochemistry*, 5th ed., Section 30.2.

48   *The muscles of a typical 150-pound adult can hold about 400 grams of glucose*: Wasserman, "Four grams of glucose," E11–E21.

48   *Any glucose beyond that is turned into fat*: Lubert Stryer, "Fatty acid metabolism," in *Biochemistry*, 5th ed. (New York: W. H. Freeman and Co., 1995), 603–28.

49   *The only thing that fructose can be stored as is fat*: Samir Softic et al., "Role of dietary fructose and hepatic de novo lipogenesis in fatty liver disease," *Digestive Diseases and Sciences* 61, no. 5 (2016): 1282–93, https://www.ncbi.nlm.nih.gov/pmc/articles/PMC4838515/.

49   *It accumulates in the liver*: Bettina Geidl-Flueck et al., "Fructose- and sucrose- but not glucose-sweetened beverages promote hepatic *de novo* lipogenesis: A randomized controlled trial," *Journal of Hepatology* 75, no. 1 (2021): 46–54, https://www.journal-of-hepatology.eu/article/S0168-8278(21)00161-6/fulltext#%20.

49   *The absence of fructose means that fewer molecules end up as fat*: João Silva et al., "Determining contributions of exogenous glucose and fructose to *de novo* fatty acid and glycerol synthesis in liver and adipose tissue," *Metabolic Engineering* 56 (2019): 69–76, https://www.sciencedirect.com/science/article/pii/S109671761930196X#fig5.

50   *The more you're able to grow the number and size of your fat cells*: Benjamin Bikman, *Why We Get Sick: The Hidden Epidemic at the Root of Most Chronic Disease and How to Fight It* (New York: BenBella, 2020).

51   *When our glycogen reserves begin to diminish, our body draws on the*

fat in our fat reserves for energy: Lubert Stryer, *Biochemistry*, 5th ed. (New York: W. H. Freeman and Co., 1995), 773–74.

51 *Weight loss is always preceded by insulin decrease*: Natasha Wiebe et al., "Temporal associations among body mass index, fasting insulin, and systemic inflammation: a systematic review and meta-analysis," *JAMA Network Open* 4, no. 3 (2021): e211263, https://jamanetwork.com/jour nals/jamanetworkopen/fullarticle/2777423.

7: FROM HEAD TO TOE

53 *Short-term symptoms associated with spikes*: Martin Picard et al., "Mitochondrial allostatic load puts the 'gluc' back in glucocorticoids," *Nature Reviews Endocrinology* 10, no. 5 (2014): 303–10, https://www .uclahealth.org/reversibility-network/workfiles/resources/publica tions/picard-endocrinol.pdf.

CONSTANT HUNGER

54 *Constant hunger*: Paula Chandler-Laney et al., "Return of hunger following a relatively high carbohydrate breakfast is associated with earlier recorded glucose peak and nadir," *Appetite* 80 (2014): 236–241, https:// www.sciencedirect.com/science/article/abs/pii/S0195666314002049.

54 *Constant hunger is a symptom of high insulin levels*: Benjamin Bikman, *Why We Get Sick: The Hidden Epidemic at the Root of Most Chronic Disease and How to Fight It* (New York: BenBella, 2020).

CRAVINGS

55 *Cravings*: Kathleen Page et al., "Circulating glucose levels modulate neural control of desire for high-calorie foods in humans," *Journal of Clinical Investigation* 121, no. 10 (2011): 4161–69, https://www.jci.org /articles/view/57873.

CHRONIC FATIGUE

56 *Chronic fatigue [. . .] people born with mitochondrial defects*: Tanja Taivassalo et al., "The spectrum of exercise tolerance in mitochondrial myopathies: a study of 40 patients," *Brain* 126, no. 2 (2003): 413–423, https://pubmed.ncbi.nlm.nih.gov/12538407/.

56 *Difficult events, whether physical or mental*: Picard, "Mitochondrial allostatic load," 303–310.

56 *Impairing the long-term ability of our mitochondria*: Picard, "Mito-chondrial allostatic load," 303–310.

56 *Diets that cause glucose roller coasters*: Kara L. Breymeyer et al., "Subjective mood and energy levels of healthy weight and overweight /obese healthy adults on high-and low-glycemic load experimental diets," *Appetite* 107 (2016): 253–259, https://pubmed.ncbi.nlm.nih.gov /27507131/.

POOR SLEEP

57 *Poor sleep*: James Gangwisch et al., "High glycemic index and glycemic load diets as risk factors for insomnia: analyses from the Women's Health Initiative," *The American Journal of Clinical Nutrition* 111, no. 2 (2020): 429–39, https://pubmed.ncbi.nlm.nih.gov/31828298/.

57 *Sleep apnea*: R. N. Aurora et al., "Obstructive Sleep Apnea and Postprandial Glucose Differences in Type 2 Diabetes Mellitus," in *A97. SRN: New Insights into the Cardiometabolic Consequences of Insufficient Sleep*, A2525–A2525, American Thoracic Society, 2020, https://www.atsjournals.org/doi/abs/10.1164/ajrccm-conference.2020.201.1 _MeetingAbstracts.A2525.

COLDS AND CORONAVIRUS COMPLICATIONS

57 *Immune system is temporarily faulty*: Nagham Jafar et al., "The effect of short-term hyperglycemia on the innate immune system," *The American Journal of the Medical Sciences* 351, no. 2 (2016): 201–ß211, https://www.amjmedsci.org/article/S0002-9629(15)00027-0/fulltext.

57 *Goodbye to five-star immune responses*: Janan Kiselar et al., "Modification of β-Defensin-2 by dicarbonyls methylglyoxal and glyoxal inhibits antibacterial and chemotactic function in vitro," *PLoS One* 10, no. 8 (2015): e0130533, https://journals.plos.org/plosone/article?id=10.1371/journal.pone.0130533.

57 *Main factors that predict whether we'll survive a coronavirus infection*: Jiaoyue Zhang et al., "Impaired fasting glucose and diabetes are related to higher risks of complications and mortality among patients with coronavirus disease 2019," *Frontiers in Endocrinology* 11 (2020): 525, https://www.frontiersin.org/articles/10.3389/fendo.2020.00525/full?report=reader.

57 *More easily infected*: Emmanuelle Logette et al., "A Machine-Generated View of the Role of Blood Glucose Levels in the Severity of COVID-19," *Frontiers in Public Health* (2021): 1068, https://www.frontiersin.org/arti

cles/10.3389/fpubh.2021.695139/full?fbclid=IwAR0RS9OVCuL9q-fb
W4gF7McCYfgRgNDQIVI4JjZE-59Sm1E7l1MFZ0ZGyoI.

57 *Twice as likely to die from the virus*: Francisco Carrasco-Sánchez et
al., "Admission hyperglycaemia as a predictor of mortality in patients
hospitalized with COVID-19 regardless of diabetes status: data from
the Spanish SEMI-COVID-19 Registry," *Annals of Medicine* 53, no. 1
(2021): 103–16, https://www.tandfonline.com/doi/full/10.1080/07853890
.2020.1836566.

GESTATIONAL DIABETES IS HARDER TO MANAGE

57 *Gestational diabetes*: Ursula Hiden et al., "Insulin and the IGF system
in the human placenta of normal and diabetic pregnancies," *Journal
of Anatomy* 215, no. 1 (2009): 60–68, https://onlinelibrary.wiley.com
/doi/full/10.1111/j.1469-7580.2008.01035.x.

57 *Insulin is responsible for encouraging growth*: Chiara Berlato et al., "Se-
lective response to insulin versus insulin-like growth factor-I and -II
and up-regulation of insulin receptor splice variant B in the differen-
tiated mouse mammary epithelium," *Endocrinology* 150, no. 6 (2009):
2924–33, https://academic.oup.com/endo/article/150/6/2924/2456369?
login=true.

58 *Mothers can reduce their likelihood of needing medication*: Carol
Major et al., "The effects of carbohydrate restriction in patients with
diet-controlled gestational diabetes," *Obstetrics & Gynecology* 91, no. 4
(1998): 600–604, https://www.sciencedirect.com/science/article/abs/pii
/S0029784498000039.

58 *Reduce the likelihood of a C-section*: Robert Moses et al., "Effect of a
low-glycemic-index diet during pregnancy on obstetric outcomes," *The
American Journal of Clinical Nutrition* 84, no. 4 (2006): 807–12, https://
academic.oup.com/ajcn/article/84/4/807/4633214.

58 *Limit their own weight gain*: James F. Clapp III et al., "Maternal carbohydrate intake and pregnancy outcome," *Proceedings of the Nutrition Society* 61, no. 1 (2002): 45–50, https://www.cambridge.org/core
/journals/proceedings-of-the-nutrition-society/article/maternal-carbo
hydrate-intake-and-pregnancy-outcome/28F8E1C5E1460E67F2F1C
E0C1D06EE81.

HOT FLASHES AND NIGHT SWEATS

58 *Hot flashes and night sweats*: Rebecca Thurston et al., "Vasomotor
symptoms and insulin resistance in the study of women's health across

the nation," *Journal of Clinical Endocrinology & Metabolism* 97, no. 10 (2012): 3487–94, https://pubmed.ncbi.nlm.nih.gov/22851488/.

58 *A 2020 study from Columbia University*: Gangwisch, "High glycemic index and glycemic load diets," 429–39.

MIGRAINE

58 *Migraine*: A. Fava et al., "Chronic migraine in women is associated with insulin resistance: a cross-sectional study," *European Journal of Neurology* 21, no. 2 (2014): 267–272, https://onlinelibrary.wiley.com /doi/abs/10.1111/ene.12289.

58 *When sufferers' insulin levels are lowered*: Cinzia Cavestro et al., "Alpha-lipoic acid shows promise to improve migraine in patients with insulin resistance: a 6-month exploratory study," *Journal of Medicinal Food* 21, no. 3 (2018): 269–73, https://www.liebertpub.com/doi /abs/10.1089/jmf.2017.0068.

MEMORY AND COGNITIVE FUNCTION

59 *Memory and cognitive function*: Rachel Ginieis et al., "The 'sweet' effect: comparative assessments of dietary sugars on cognitive performance," *Physiology & Behavior* 184 (2018): 242–47, https://pubmed .ncbi.nlm.nih.gov/29225094/.

59 *Worst first thing in the morning*: Ginieis, "The 'sweet' effect," 242–47.

ACNE AND OTHER SKIN CONDITIONS

60 *Acne and other skin conditions*: Hyuck Hoon Kwon et al., "Clinical and histological effect of a low glycaemic load diet in treatment of acne vulgaris in Korean patients: a randomized, controlled trial," *Acta Dermato Venereologica* 92, no. 3 (2012): 241–46, https://pubmed.ncbi.nlm .nih.gov/22678562/.

60 *Acne clears up*: Robyn N. Smith et al., "A low-glycemic-load diet improves symptoms in acne vulgaris patients: a randomized controlled trial," *The American Journal of Clinical Nutrition* 86, no. 1 (2007): 107–15, https://pubmed.ncbi.nlm.nih.gov/17616769/.

AGING AND ARTHRITIS

60 *The more often we spike, the faster we age*: George Suji et al., "Glucose, glycation and aging," *Biogerontology* 5, no. 6 (2004): 365–73, https:// link.springer.com/article/10.1007/s10522-004-3189-0.

60 *Glycation, free radicals, and the subsequent inflammation*: Roma

Pahwa et al., "Chronic Inflammation," (2018), https://www.ncbi.nlm.nih.gov/books/NBK493173/.

60 *Rheumatoid arthritis*: Pahwa, "Chronic Inflammation."

60 *Degradation of cartilage*: Robert A. Greenwald et al., "Inhibition of collagen gelation by action of the superoxide radical," *Arthritis & Rheumatism: Official Journal of the American College of Rheumatology* 22, no. 3 (1979): 251–59, https://pubmed.ncbi.nlm.nih.gov/217393/.

61 *Osteoarthritis*: Biplab Giri et al., "Chronic hyperglycemia mediated physiological alteration and metabolic distortion leads to organ dysfunction, infection, cancer progression and other pathophysiological consequences: an update on glucose toxicity," *Biomedicine & Pharmacotherapy*, no. 107 (2018): 306–328, https://www.sciencedirect.com/science/article/abs/pii/S0753332218322406.

61 *Our bones waste away*: John Tower, "Programmed cell death in aging," *Ageing Research Reviews* 23 (2015): 90–100, https://www.ncbi.nlm.nih.gov/pmc/articles/PMC4480161/.

ALZHEIMER'S AND DEMENTIA

61 *Brain is vulnerable to the consequences*: Charles Watt et al., "Glycemic variability and CNS inflammation: Reviewing the connection," *Nutrients* 12, no. 12 (2020): 3906, https://pubmed.ncbi.nlm.nih.gov/33371247/.

61 *Key factor in almost all chronic degenerative diseases*: Pahwa, "Chronic Inflammation."

61 *Alzheimer's is sometimes called "type 3 diabetes"*: Suzanne M. De La Monte et al., "Alzheimer's disease is type 3 diabetes—evidence reviewed," *Journal of Diabetes Science and Technology* 2, no. 6 (2008): 1101–13, https://journals.sagepub.com/doi/abs/10.1177/193229680800200619.

61 *Type 2 diabetes are four times more likely to develop Alzheimer's*: Robert H. Lustig, *Metabolical: The Lure and the Lies of Processed Food, Nutrition, and Modern Medicine* (New York: Harper Wave, 2021).

61 *The signs are visible early, too*: Jiyin Zhou et al., "Diabetic cognitive dysfunction: from bench to clinic," *Current Medicinal Chemistry* 27, no. 19 (2020): 3151–67, https://pubmed.ncbi.nlm.nih.gov/30727866/.

61 *The signs are visible early, too*: Auriel A. Willette et al., "Association of insulin resistance with cerebral glucose uptake in late middle–aged adults at risk for Alzheimer disease," *JAMA Neurology* 72, no. 9 (2015): 1013–20, https://pubmed.ncbi.nlm.nih.gov/26214150/.

61 *The signs are visible early, too*: Christine M. Burns et al., "Higher serum glucose levels are associated with cerebral hypometabolism in Alzheimer regions," *Neurology* 80, no. 17 (2013): 1557–64, https://www.ncbi.nlm.nih.gov/pmc/articles/PMC3662330/.

61 *Studies show short-term*: Mark A. Reger et al., "Effects of ß-hydroxybutyrate on cognition in memory-impaired adults," *Neurobiology of Aging* 25, no. 3 (2004): 311–14, https://www.sciencedirect.com/science/article/abs/pii/S0197458003000873.

61 *And long-term improvements*: Dale E. Bredesen et al., "Reversal of cognitive decline: a novel therapeutic program," *Aging* (Albany, NY) 6, no. 9 (2014): 707, https://www.ncbi.nlm.nih.gov/pmc/articles/PMC4221920/.

61 *A therapeutic program out of UCLA*: Bredesen, "Reversal of cognitive decline," 707.

CANCER RISK

62 *Cancer risk*: Amar S. Ahmad et al., "Trends in the lifetime risk of developing cancer in Great Britain: comparison of risk for those born from 1930 to 1960," *British Journal of Cancer* 112, no. 5 (2015): 943–47, https://www.nature.com/articles/bjc2014606.

62 *Poor diet, together with smoking, is the main driver*: Lustig, *Metabolical*.

62 *Cancer may begin with*: Florian R. Greten et al., "Inflammation and cancer: triggers, mechanisms, and consequences," *Immunity* 51, no. 1 (2019): 27–41, https://www.sciencedirect.com/science/article/pii/S10747 6131930295X.

62 *When there is more insulin present, cancer spreads even faster*: Rachel J. Perry et al., "Mechanistic links between obesity, insulin, and cancer," *Trends in Cancer* 6, no. 2 (2020): 75–78, https://www.sciencedirect.com/science/article/abs/pii/S2405803319302614.

62 *Glucose is the key to many of these processes*: Tetsuro Tsujimoto et al., "Association between hyperinsulinemia and increased risk of cancer death in nonobese and obese people: A population-based observational study," *International Journal of Cancer* 141, no. 1 (2017): 102–111, https://onlinelibrary.wiley.com/doi/full/10.1002/ijc.30729.

DEPRESSIVE EPISODES

62 *Depressive episodes*: Breymeyer, "Subjective mood and energy levels," 253–59.

62 *Worsening moods, more depressive symptoms*: Rachel A. Cheatham

et al., "Long-term effects of provided low and high glycemic load low energy diets on mood and cognition," *Physiology & Behavior* 98, no. 3 (2009): 374–79, https://pubmed.ncbi.nlm.nih.gov/19576915/.

62   *Worsening moods, more depressive symptoms*: Sue Penckofer et al., "Does glycemic variability impact mood and quality of life?" *Diabetes, Technology & Therapeutics* 14, no. 4 (2012): 303–10, https://www.ncbi .nlm.nih.gov/pmc/articles/PMC3317401/.

62   *Symptoms get worse as the spikes get more extreme*: James E. Gangwisch et al., "High glycemic index diet as a risk factor for depression: analyses from the Women's Health Initiative," *The American Journal of Clinical Nutrition* 102, no. 2 (2015): 454–63, https://www.ncbi.nlm .nih.gov/pmc/articles/PMC4515860/.

GUT ISSUES

63   *High glucose levels could increase leaky gut syndrome*: Fernando F. Anhê et al., "Glucose alters the symbiotic relationships between gut microbiota and host physiology," *American Journal of Physiology-Endocrinology and Metabolism* 318, no. 2 (2020): E111–E116, https:// pubmed.ncbi.nlm.nih.gov/31794261/.

63   *Food allergies and other autoimmune diseases*: Lustig, *Metabolical*.

63   *Can get rid of their heartburn or acid reflux*: William S. Yancy et al., "Improvements of gastroesophageal reflux disease after initiation of a low-carbohydrate diet: Five brief case reports," *Alternative Therapies in Health and Medicine* 7, no. 6 (2001): 120, https://search.proquest.com /openview/1c418d7f0548f58a5c647b1204d3f6a7/1?pq-origsite=gscholar &cbl=32528.

63   *Gut health is linked to mental health*: Jessica M. Yano et al., "Indigenous bacteria from the gut microbiota regulate host serotonin biosynthesis," *Cell* 161, no. 2 (2015): 264–76, https://www.ncbi.nlm.nih.gov /pmc/articles/PMC4393509/.

63   *Gut health is linked to mental health*: Roberto Mazzoli et al., "The neuro-endocrinological role of microbial glutamate and GABA signaling," *Frontiers in Microbiology* 7 (2016): 1934, https://www.ncbi.nlm .nih.gov/pmc/articles/PMC5127831/.

63   *The gut and the brain are connected*: Emeran A. Mayer, "Gut feelings: the emerging biology of gut-brain communication," *Nature Reviews Neuroscience* 12, no. 8 (2011): 453–66, https://www.ncbi.nlm.nih .gov/pmc/articles/PMC3845678/.

63   *Information is sent back and forth between them*: Sigrid Breit et al.,

"Vagus nerve as modulator of the brain–gut axis in psychiatric and inflammatory disorders," *Frontiers in Psychiatry* 9 (2018): 44, https://www.ncbi.nlm.nih.gov/pubmed/29593576.

63　*Information is sent back and forth between them*: Bruno Bonaz et al., "The vagus nerve at the interface of the microbiota-gut-brain axis," *Frontiers in Neuroscience* 12 (2018): 49, https://www.ncbi.nlm.nih.gov/pubmed/29467611.

HEART DISEASE

63　*Half the people who have a heart attack have* normal *levels of cholesterol*: Michael D. Miedema et al., "Statin eligibility and outpatient care prior to ST-segment elevation myocardial infarction," *Journal of the American Heart Association* 6, no. 4 (2017): e005333, https://www.ahajournals.org/doi/10.1161/JAHA.116.005333.

64　*Our liver starts producing LDL pattern B*: Bikman, *Why We Get Sick*.

64　*If and when that cholesterol is oxidized*: Bikman, *Why We Get Sick*.

64　*Each additional glucose* spike *increases our risk of dying of a heart attack*: Koichi Node et al., "Postprandial hyperglycemia as an etiological factor in vascular failure," *Cardiovascular Diabetology* 8, no. 1 (2009): 1–10, https://pubmed.ncbi.nlm.nih.gov/19402896/.

64　*Each additional glucose* spike *increases our risk of dying of a heart attack*: Antonio Ceriello et al., "Oscillating glucose is more deleterious to endothelial function and oxidative stress than mean glucose in normal and type 2 diabetic patients," *Diabetes* 57, no. 5 (2008): 1349–54, https://pubmed.ncbi.nlm.nih.gov/18299315/.

64　*Each additional glucose* spike *increases our risk of dying of a heart attack*: Michelle Flynn et al., "Transient intermittent hyperglycemia accelerates atherosclerosis by promoting myelopoiesis," *Circulation Research* 127, no. 7 (2020): 877–92, https://www.ahajournals.org/doi/full/10.1161/CIRCRESAHA.120.316653.

64　*Each additional glucose* spike *increases our risk of dying of a heart attack*: E. Succurro et al., "Elevated one-hour post-load plasma glucose levels identifies subjects with normal glucose tolerance but early carotid atherosclerosis," *Atherosclerosis* 207, no. 1 (2009): 245–49, https://www.sciencedirect.com/science/article/abs/pii/S0021915009002718.

64　*Statins lower LDL pattern A*: Bikman, *Why We Get Sick*.

64　*Statins don't decrease the risk of a first heart attack*: Lustig, *Metabolical*.

65　*A ratio that is surprisingly accurate in predicting LDL size*: Bikman, *Why We Get Sick*.

65   *Measuring C-reactive protein*: Paul M. Ridker et al., "Comparison of C-reactive protein and low-density lipoprotein cholesterol levels in the prediction of first cardiovascular events," *New England Journal of Medicine* 347, no. 20 (2002): 1557–65, https://www.nejm.org/doi/full/10.1056/NEJMoa021993.

INFERTILITY AND POLYCYSTIC OVARIAN SYNDROME (PCOS)

65   *Women and men with high insulin levels are more likely to be infertile*: Tetsurou Sakumoto et al., "Insulin resistance/hyperinsulinemia and reproductive disorders in infertile women," *Reproductive Medicine and Biology* 9, no. 4 (2010): 185–90, https://www.ncbi.nlm.nih.gov/pmc/articles/PMC5904600/.

65   *Women and men with high insulin levels are more likely to be infertile*: LaTasha B. Craig et al., "Increased prevalence of insulin resistance in women with a history of recurrent pregnancy loss," *Fertility and Sterility* 78, no. 3 (2002): 487–490, https://www.sciencedirect.com/science/article/abs/pii/S0015028202032478.

65   *Women and men with high insulin levels are more likely to be infertile*: Nelly Pitteloud et al., "Increasing insulin resistance is associated with a decrease in Leydig cell testosterone secretion in men," *Journal of Clinical Endocrinology & Metabolism* 90, no. 5 (2005): 2636–41, https://academic.oup.com/jcem/article/90/5/2636/2836773.

65   *The more glucose spikes in our diet*: Jorge E. Chavarro et al., "A prospective study of dietary carbohydrate quantity and quality in relation to risk of ovulatory infertility," *European Journal of Clinical Nutrition* 63, no. 1 (2009): 78–86, https://www.ncbi.nlm.nih.gov/pmc/articles/PMC3066074/.

65   *Polycystic ovarian syndrome (PCOS)*: Centers for Disease Control and Prevention, "PCOS (Polycystic Ovary Syndrome) and Diabetes," CDC, accessed August 30, 2021, https://www.cdc.gov/diabetes/basics/pcos.html.

65   *Insulin tells the ovaries to produce more testosterone*: John E. Nestler et al., "Insulin stimulates testosterone biosynthesis by human thecal cells from women with polycystic ovary syndrome by activating its own receptor and using inositolglycan mediators as the signal transduction system," *Journal of Clinical Endocrinology & Metabolism* 83, no. 6 (1998): 2001–2005, https://academic.oup.com/jcem/article/83/6/2001/2865383?login=true.

65   *On top of that, with too much insulin*: Bikman, *Why We Get Sick*.

65 *Women suffering from PCOS display masculine traits*: CDC, "PCOS."

66 *In a study performed at Duke University*: John C. Mavropoulos et al., "The effects of a low-carbohydrate, ketogenic diet on the polycystic ovary syndrome: a pilot study," *Nutrition & Metabolism* 2, no. 1 (2005): 1–5, https://www.ncbi.nlm.nih.gov/pmc/articles/PMC1334192/.

66 *For men, dysregulated glucose is also linked to infertility*: Zeeshan Anwar et al., "Erectile dysfunction: An underestimated presentation in patients with diabetes mellitus," *Indian Journal of Psychological Medicine* 39, no. 5 (2017): 600–604, https://www.ncbi.nlm.nih.gov/pmc/articles/PMC5688886/.

66 *Erectile dysfunction in men under 40 years*: Fengjuan Yao et al., "Erectile dysfunction may be the first clinical sign of insulin resistance and endothelial dysfunction in young men," *Clinical Research in Cardiology* 102, no. 9 (2013): 645–51, https://link.springer.com/article/10.1007/s00392-013-0577-y.

INSULIN RESISTANCE AND TYPE 2 DIABETES

66 *Type 2 diabetes is a global epidemic*: Sudesna Chatterjee et al., "Type 2 diabetes," *The Lancet* 389, no. 10085 (2017): 2239–2251, https://www.sciencedirect.com/science/article/abs/pii/S0140673617300582.

67 *More inflammation, a process set off by glucose spikes, makes it worse*: Marc Y. Donath et al., "Type 2 diabetes as an inflammatory disease," *Nature Reviews Immunology* 11, no. 2 (2011): 98–107, https://pubmed.ncbi.nlm.nih.gov/21233852/.

68 *Most effective way to reverse type 2 diabetes is to flatten our glucose curves*: Joshua Z. Goldenberg et al., "Efficacy and safety of low and very low carbohydrate diets for type 2 diabetes remission: systematic review and meta-analysis of published and unpublished randomized trial data," *BMJ* 372 (2021), https://www.bmj.com/content/372/bmj.m4743.

68 *In one study, type 2 diabetics*: William S. Yancy et al., "A low-carbohydrate, ketogenic diet to treat type 2 diabetes," *Nutrition & Metabolism* 2, no. 1 (2005): 1–7, https://link.springer.com/article/10.1186/1743-7075-2-34.

68 *American Diabetes Association (the ADA) started endorsing glucose-flattening diets*: Alison B. Evert et al., "Nutrition therapy for adults with diabetes or prediabetes: a consensus report," *Diabetes Care* 42, no. 5 (2019): 731–54, https://care.diabetesjournals.org/content/diacare/early/2019/04/10/dci19-0014.full.pdf.

NONALCOHOLIC FATTY LIVER DISEASE

68 *Excess fructose could cause liver disease*: Robert H. Lustig, "Fructose: it's 'alcohol without the buzz,'" *Advances in Nutrition* 4, no. 2 (2013): 226–35, https://www.ncbi.nlm.nih.gov/pmc/articles/PMC3649103/.

68 *One out of every four adults has NAFLD*: Zobair M. Younossi et al., "Global epidemiology of nonalcoholic fatty liver disease—meta-analytic assessment of prevalence, incidence, and outcomes," *Hepatology* 64, no. 1 (2016): 73–84, https://aasldpubs.onlinelibrary.wiley.com/doi/full/10.1002/hep.28431.

68 *In people who are overweight, it's even more common*: Ruth C. R. Meex et al., "Hepatokines: linking nonalcoholic fatty liver disease and insulin resistance," *Nature Reviews Endocrinology* 13, no. 9 (2017): 509–20, https://www.nature.com/articles/nrendo.2017.56.

WRINKLES AND CATARACTS

69 *Broken collagen leads to sagging skin and wrinkles*: F. William Danby, "Nutrition and aging skin: sugar and glycation," *Clinics in Dermatology* 28, no. 4 (2010): 409–411, https://www.sciencedirect.com/science/article/abs/pii/S0738081X10000428.

69 *The more glycation, the more*: Paraskevi Gkogkolou et al., "Advanced glycation end products: key players in skin aging?" *Dermato-endocrinology* 4, no. 3 (2012): 259–70, https://www.ncbi.nlm.nih.gov/pmc/articles/PMC3583887/.

69 *We develop cataracts*: Ashok V. Katta et al., "Glycation of lens crystalline protein in the pathogenesis of various forms of cataract," *Biomedical Research* 20, no. 2 (2009): 119–21, https://www.researchgate.net/profile/Ashok-Katta-3/publication/233419577_Glycation_of_lens_crystalline_protein_in_the_pathogenesis_of_various_forms_of_cataract/links/02e7e531342066c955000000/Glycation-of-lens-crystalline-protein-in-the-pathogenesis-of-various-forms-of-cataract.pdf.

70 *Odds are, you are among the 88 percent of adults who have dysregulated glucose levels*: Joana Araújo et al., "Prevalence of optimal metabolic health in American adults: National Health and Nutrition Examination Survey 2009–2016," *Metabolic Syndrome and Related Disorders* 17, no. 1 (2019): 46–52, https://www.liebertpub.com/doi/10.1089/met.2018.0105.

HACK 1: EAT FOODS IN THE RIGHT ORDER

73   *If you eat the items of a meal containing starch, fiber, sugar, protein, and fat in a specific order*: Alpana P. Shukla et al., "Food order has a significant impact on postprandial glucose and insulin levels," *Diabetes Care* 38, no. 7 (2015): e98–e99, https://care.diabetesjournals.org/content /38/7/e98.

73   *This is true for anyone, with or without diabetes*: Kimiko Nishino et al., "Consuming carbohydrates after meat or vegetables lowers postprandial excursions of glucose and insulin in nondiabetic subjects," *Journal of Nutritional Science and Vitaminology* 64, no. 5 (2018): 316–20, https://www.researchgate.net/publication/328640463_Consuming_ Carbohydrates_after_Meat_or_Vegetables_Lowers_Postprandial_Ex cursions_of_Glucose_and_Insulin_in_Nondiabetic_Subjects.

73   *The effect of this sequencing is comparable to the effects of diabetes medications*: Shukla, "Food order has a significant impact," e98–e99.

73   *A startling study from 2016 proved the finding even more definitively*: Domenico Tricò et al., "Manipulating the sequence of food ingestion improves glycemic control in type 2 diabetic patients under free-living conditions," *Nutrition & Diabetes* 6, no. 8 (2016): e226, https://www.na ture.com/articles/nutd201633/.

74   *About three calories' worth of food trickles through*: Diana Gentilcore et al., "Effects of fat on gastric emptying of and the glycemic, insulin, and incretin responses to a carbohydrate meal in type 2 diabetes," *Journal of Clinical Endocrinology & Metabolism* 91, no. 6 (2006): 2062–67, https://academic.oup.com/jcem/article/91/6/2062/2843371?login =true.

75   *Fiber has three superpowers*: J. R. Perry et al., "A review of physiological effects of soluble and insoluble dietary fibers," *Journal of Nutrition and Food Sciences* 6, no. 2 (2016): 476, https://www.longdom.org /open-access/a-review-of-physiological-effects-of-soluble-and-insolu ble-dietary-fibers-2155-9600-1000476.pdf.

76   *Foods containing fat also slow down gastric emptying*: Gentilcore, "Effects of fat on gastric emptying," 2062–67.

79   *When we eat foods in the right order, our pancreas produces less insulin*: Shukla, "Food order has a significant impact," e98–e99.

79   *When we eat foods in the right order, our pancreas produces less insulin*: Nishino, "Consuming carbohydrates," 316–20.

82   *Ghrelin stays suppressed for much longer*: Alpana P. Shukla et al.,

"Effect of food order on ghrelin suppression," *Diabetes Care* 41, no. 5 (2018): e76–e77, https://care.diabetesjournals.org/content/41/5/e76.

83 *Research also shows that in postmenopausal women*: James E. Gangwisch et al., "High glycemic index and glycemic load diets as risk factors for insomnia: analyses from the Women's Health Initiative," *The American Journal of Clinical Nutrition* 111, no. 2 (2020): 429–39, https://pubmed.ncbi.nlm.nih.gov/31828298/.

83 *"Float on top of the contents of the stomach and eventually putrefy"*: David Gentilcore, *Food and Health in Early Modern Europe: Diet, Medicine and Society 1450–1800* (New York: Bloomsbury Publishing, 2015).

85 *Second, our stomach is an acidic environment*: R. H. Hunt et al., "The stomach in health and disease," *Gut* 64, no. 10 (2015): 1650–68, https://www.ncbi.nlm.nih.gov/pmc/articles/PMC4835810/.

85 *Nothing can rot in the stomach*: Hunt, "The stomach in health and disease," 1650–68.

85 *In Roman times, a meal generally started with*: Patrick Faas, *Around the Roman Table: Food and Feasting in Ancient Rome* (Chicago: University of Chicago Press, 2005).

HACK 2: ADD A GREEN STARTER TO ALL YOUR MEALS

91 *The amount of fiber we eat these days is much lower*: Diane Quagliani et al., "Closing America's fiber intake gap: communication strategies from a food and fiber summit," *American Journal of Lifestyle Medicine* 11, no. 1 (2017): 80–85, https://www.ncbi.nlm.nih.gov/pmc/articles/PMC6124841/.

91 *"Nutrient of public health concern"*: United States Dietary Guidelines Advisory Committee, "Dietary guidelines for Americans, 2010," no. 232.

92 *This plant-made substance is incredibly important to us*: Thomas M. Barber et al., "The health benefits of dietary fibre," *Nutrients* 12, no. 10 (2020): 3209, https://www.mdpi.com/2072-6643/12/10/3209/pdf.

92 *It creates a viscous mesh in our intestine*: Martin O. Weickert et al., "Metabolic effects of dietary fiber consumption and prevention of diabetes," *Journal of Nutrition* 138, no. 3 (2008): 439–42, https://academic.oup.com/jn/article/138/3/439/4670214.

92 *The additional fiber reduced the glucose spike of the bread*: Jannie Yi Fang Yang et al., "The effects of functional fiber on postprandial glycemia, energy intake, satiety, palatability and gastrointestinal wellbeing: a randomized crossover trial," *Nutrition Journal* 13, no. 1

(2014): 1–9, https://nutritionj.biomedcentral.com/articles/10.1186/14 75-2891-13-76.

94   *With a flatter curve, we stay full longer*: Paula C. Chandler-Laney et al., "Return of hunger following a relatively high carbohydrate breakfast is associated with earlier recorded glucose peak and nadir," *Appetite* 80 (2014):236–41,https://www.sciencedirect.com/science/article/abs/pii/S0 195666314002049.

94   *Avoid the glucose dip that leads to cravings*: Patrick Wyatt et al., "Post-prandial glycaemic dips predict appetite and energy intake in healthy individuals," *Nature Metabolism* 3, no. 4 (2021): 523–29, https://www .nature.com/articles/s42255-021-00383-x.

100 *A fiber supplement at the beginning of a meal can help*: Lorenzo Nesti et al., "Impact of nutrient type and sequence on glucose tolerance: Physiological insights and therapeutic implications," *Frontiers in Endocrinology* 10 (2019): 144, https://www.frontiersin.org/articles/10.3389 /fendo.2019.00144/full#B58.

101 *Diabetes isn't just about genes*: Michael Multhaup et al., *The Science Behind 23andMe's Type 2 Diabetes Report*, 2019, accessed August 30, 2021, https://permalinks.23andme.com/pdf/23_19-Type2Diabetes_March 2019.pdf.

101 *Our lifestyle is still the main reason we do—or don't*: Michael E. J. Lean et al., "Primary care-led weight management for remission of type 2 diabetes (DiRECT): an open-label, cluster-randomised trial," *The Lancet* 391, no. 10120 (2018): 541–51, https://pubmed.ncbi.nlm.nih .gov/29221645/.

HACK 3: STOP COUNTING CALORIES

104 *In 2015, a research team out of UC San Francisco proved that*: Robert H. Lustig et al., "Isocaloric fructose restriction and metabolic improvement in children with obesity and metabolic syndrome," *Obesity* 24, no. 2 (2016): 453–60, https://onlinelibrary.wiley.com/doi/full/10.1002 /oby.21371.

105 *People who focus on flattening their glucose curves can eat* more *calories*: Laura R. Saslow et al., "Twelve-month outcomes of a randomized trial of a moderate-carbohydrate versus very low-carbohydrate diet in overweight adults with type 2 diabetes mellitus or prediabetes," *Nutrition & Diabetes* 7, no. 12 (2017): 1–6, https://www.nature.com/articles /s41387-017-0006-9.

106 *A 2017 study from the University of Michigan*: Saslow, "Twelve-month outcomes," 1–6.

107 *Insulin reduction is primordial and always precedes weight loss*: Natasha Wiebe et al., "Temporal associations among body mass index, fasting insulin, and systemic inflammation: a systematic review and meta-analysis," *JAMA Network Open* 4, no. 3 (2021): e211263, https://jama network.com/journals/jamanetworkopen/fullarticle/2777423.

107 *We can completely ignore calories and still lose weight*: Tian Hu et al., "Adherence to low-carbohydrate and low-fat diets in relation to weight loss and cardiovascular risk factors," *Obesity Science & Practice* 2, no. 1 (2016): 24–31, https://onlinelibrary.wiley.com/doi/full/10.1002/osp4.23.

109 *Reactive hypoglycemia is a common condition*: Hanne Mumm et al., "Prevalence and possible mechanisms of reactive hypoglycemia in polycystic ovary syndrome," *Human Reproduction* 31, no. 5 (2016): 1105–12, https://pubmed.ncbi.nlm.nih.gov/27008892/.

109 *Their glucose level can get so low that it causes a coma*: Gita Shafiee et al., "The importance of hypoglycemia in diabetic patients," *Journal of Diabetes & Metabolic Disorders* 11, no. 1 (2012): 1–7, https://link .springer.com/article/10.1186/2251-6581-11-17.

109 *The greater the dip, the more hungry we become*: Wyatt, "Postprandial glycaemic dips," 523–29.

HACK 4: FLATTEN YOUR BREAKFAST CURVE

117 *Twenty participants were recruited, both men and women*: Heather Hall et al., "Glucotypes reveal new patterns of glucose dysregulation," *PLoS Biology* 16, no. 7 (2018): e2005143, https://pubmed.ncbi.nlm.nih .gov/30040822/.

118 *2.7 billion boxes of cereal are sold every year*: Statista report based on the U.S. Census data and Simmons National Consumer Survey (NHCS).

118 *Contains three times as much sugar as the cereal*: Nutritionix Grocery Database, "Honey Nut Cheerios, Cereal," Nutritionix, accessed August 30, 2021, https://www.nutritionix.com/i/general-mills/honey-nut-cheer ios-cereal/51d2fb6dcc9bff111580dc91.

118 *When 60 million Americans eat a cereal such as*: Statista report based on the U.S. Census data and Simmons National Consumer Survey (NHCS).

119 *One with more carbohydrates leads to less available circulating energy*:

Kim J. Shimy et al., "Effects of dietary carbohydrate content on circulating metabolic fuel availability in the postprandial state," *Journal of the Endocrine Society* 4, no. 7 (2020): bvaa062, https://academic.oup.com/jes/article/4/7/bvaa062/5846215.

120 *A breakfast that creates a big glucose spike*: Chandler-Laney, "Return of hunger," 236–41.

120 *That breakfast will deregulate our glucose levels for the rest of the day*: Courtney R. Chang et al., "Restricting carbohydrates at breakfast is sufficient to reduce 24-hour exposure to postprandial hyperglycemia and improve glycemic variability," *The American Journal of Clinical Nutrition* 109, no. 5 (2019): 1302–09, https://academic.oup.com/ajcn/article/109/5/1302/5435774?login=true.

120 *A flat breakfast, on the other hand*: Chang, "Restricting carbohydrates at breakfast," 1302–1309.

122 *A century ago, the California Fruit Growers Exchange*: Adee Braun, "Misunderstanding Orange Juice as a Health Drink," *The Atlantic*, 2014, https://www.theatlantic.com/health/archive/2014/02/misunderstanding-orange-juice-as-a-health-drink/283579/.

123 *By blending a piece of fruit, we pulverise the fiber*: KeXue Zhu et al., "Effect of ultrafine grinding on hydration and antioxidant properties of wheat bran dietary fiber," *Food Research International* 43, no. 4 (2010): 943–48, https://www.sciencedirect.com/science/article/abs/pii/S0963996910000232.

123 *One bottle of orange juice*: U.S. Department of Agriculture, "Tropicana Pure Premium Antioxidant Advantage No Pulp Orange Juice 59 Fluid Ounce Plastic Bottle," FoodData Central, 2019, accessed August 30, 2019, https://fdc.nal.usda.gov/fdc-app.html#/food-details/762958/nutrients.

123 *That's the concentrated sugar of three whole oranges*: U.S. Department of Agriculture, "Oranges, raw, navels," FoodData Central, 2019, accessed August 30, 2019, https://fdc.nal.usda.gov/fdc-app.html#/food-details/746771/nutrients.

123 *It's the same amount of sugar as in a can of Coca-Cola*: U.S. Department of Agriculture, "Coca-Cola Life Can, 12 fl oz," FoodData Central, 2019, accessed August 30, 2019, https://fdc.nal.usda.gov/fdc-app.html#/food-details/771674/nutrients.

123 *With just one bottle of orange juice*: American Heart Association, "Added Sugars," Heart, accessed August 30, 2019, https://www.heart.org/en/healthy-living/healthy-eating/eat-smart/sugar/added-sugars.

128   *And the answer to whether sugar makes your brain work better is . . . no*:
      Rachel Galioto et al., "The effects of breakfast and breakfast composi-
      tion on cognition in adults," *Advances in Nutrition* 7, no. 3 (2016): 576S–
      89S, https://academic.oup.com/advances/article/7/3/576S/4558060.

136   *Research shows that when people with type 2 diabetes replace their
      oatmeal*: Martha Nydia Ballesteros et al., "One egg per day improves
      inflammation when compared to an oatmeal-based breakfast without
      increasing other cardiometabolic risk factors in diabetic patients," *Nutri-
      ents* 7, no. 5 (2015): 3449–63, https://www.mdpi.com/2072-6643/7/5/3449.

HACK 5: HAVE ANY TYPE OF SUGAR YOU LIKE—THEY'RE ALL THE SAME

138   *And misinformation is rampant*: Republic of the Philippines Depart-
      ment of Science and Technology, "Glycemic Index of Coco Sugar,"
      Internet Archive, accessed August 30, 2019, https://web.archive.org
      /web/20131208042347/http://www.pca.da.gov.ph/pdf/glycemic.pdf.

138   *And that was later proven to be wrong*: University of Sydney Glyce-
      mic Index Research Service, "Glycemic Index of Coconut Sugar,"
      Glycemic Index, accessed August 30, 2021, https://glycemicindex.com
      /foodSearch.php?num=2659&ak=detail.

142   *Fructose is worse for us than glucose*: Robert H. Lustig, "Fructose: it's
      'alcohol without the buzz'," *Advances in Nutrition* 4, no. 2 (2013): 226–
      235, https://www.ncbi.nlm.nih.gov/pmc/articles/PMC3649103/.

143   *And fun fact, there aren't that many antioxidants in honey*: There are
      5.15 mg/kg of flavonoids as antioxidants in multi-floral honey. One
      teaspoon is 4 grams. That gives 0.02 mg of flavonoids per teaspoon of
      honey. Goran Šarića et al., "The changes of flavonoids in honey during
      storage," *Processes* 8, no. 8 (2020): 943, https://www.mdpi.com/2227
      -9717/8/8/943/pdf: 100 grams of blueberries contains on average 4 mg
      of flavonoids. One blueberry is about 1 gram. That's 0.04 mg per blue-
      berry. Sonia de Pascual-Teresa et al., "Flavanols and anthocyanins in
      cardiovascular health: a review of current evidence," *International
      Journal of Molecular Sciences* 11, no. 4 (2010): 1679–1703, https://www
      .researchgate.net/publication/44609005_Flavanols_and_Anthocya
      nins_in_Cardiovascular_Health_A_Review_of_Current_Evidence.

144   *When people switch from drinking diet sodas*: A. Madjd et al., "Ef-
      fects of replacing diet beverages with water on weight loss and weight

maintenance: 18-month follow-up, randomized clinical trial," *International Journal of Obesity* 42, no. 4 (2018): 835–840, https://www.nature.com/articles/ijo2017306.

145 *What's more, preliminary studies suggest*: J. E. Blundell et al., "Paradoxical effects of an intense sweetener (aspartame) on appetite," *The Lancet (USA)* (1986), https://agris.fao.org/agris-search/search.do?recordID=US8731275.

146 *The theory posits further that*: Susan E. Swithers et al., "A role for sweet taste: calorie predictive relations in energy regulation by rats," *Behavioral Neuroscience* 122, no. 1 (2008): 161, https://psycnet.apa.org/doiLanding?doi=10.1037%2F0735-7044.122.1.161.

146 *Artificial sweeteners may also change the composition of our intestinal bacteria*: Francisco Javier Ruiz-Ojeda et al., "Effects of sweeteners on the gut microbiota: a review of experimental studies and clinical trials," *Advances in Nutrition* 10, no. suppl_1 (2019): S31–S48, https://www.ncbi.nlm.nih.gov/pmc/articles/PMC6363527/.

146 *There are some artificial sweeteners I'd recommend you avoid*: Stephen D. Anton et al., "Effects of stevia, aspartame, and sucrose on food intake, satiety, and postprandial glucose and insulin levels," *Appetite* 55, no. 1 (2010): 37–43, https://www.sciencedirect.com/science/article/abs/pii/S0195666310000826.

HACK 6: PICK DESSERT OVER A SWEET SNACK

149 *They keep working for* four hours *on average after our last bite*: Louis Monnier et al., "Target for glycemic control: concentrating on glucose," *Diabetes Care* 32, no. suppl 2 (2009): S199–S204, https://www.ncbi.nlm.nih.gov/pmc/articles/PMC2811454/.

149 *The postprandial state is the period of our day*: Maarten R. Soeters, "Food intake sequence modulates postprandial glycemia," *Clinical Nutrition* 39, no. 8 (2020): 2335–36, https://www.clinicalnutritionjournal.com/article/S0261-5614(20)30299-5/abstract.

149 *To digest, sort, and store the molecules*: Nagham Jafar et al., "The effect of short-term hyperglycemia on the innate immune system," *The American Journal of the Medical Sciences* 351, no. 2 (2016): 201–11, https://www.amjmedsci.org/article/S0002-9629(15)00027-0/fulltext.

149 *Insulin levels, oxidative stress, and inflammation increase*: Amber M. Milan et al., "Comparisons of the postprandial inflammatory and endotoxaemic responses to mixed meals in young and older individuals:

a randomised trial," *Nutrients* 9, no. 4 (2017): 354, https://www.ncbi.nlm
.nih.gov/pmc/articles/PMC5409693/.

149   *We tend to spend about 20 hours*: Barry M. Popkin et al., "Does hun-
      ger and satiety drive eating anymore? Increasing eating occasions and
      decreasing time between eating occasions in the United States," *The
      American Journal of Clinical Nutrition* 91, no. 5 (2010): 1342–47, https://
      academic.oup.com/ajcn/article/91/5/1342/4597335?login=true.

149   *Up through the 1980s, people didn't snack*: Popkin, "Does hunger and
      satiety drive eating anymore?" 1342–47.

150   *Our organs are on cleanup duty*: M. Ribeiro et al., "Insulin decreases
      autophagy and leads to cartilage degradation," *Osteoarthritis and Car-
      tilage* 24, no. 4 (2016): 731–739, https://www.sciencedirect.com/science
      /article/pii/S1063458415013709#.

150   *The gurgling we feel in our small intestine*: Giulia Enders, *Gut: The In-
      side Story of Our Body's Most Underrated Organ* (rev. ed.) (Vancouver:
      Greystone Books Ltd., 2018).

150   *Scientists in the Czech Republic, in 2014, tested this*: Hana Kahleova et
      al., "Eating two larger meals a day (breakfast and lunch) is more effec-
      tive than six smaller meals in a reduced-energy regimen for patients
      with type 2 diabetes: a randomised crossover study," *Diabetologia* 57,
      no. 8 (2014): 1552–60, https://link.springer.com/article/10.1007/s00125
      -014-3253-5.

154   *The benefits are more pronounced for men*: Leonie K. Heilbronn et al.,
      "Glucose tolerance and skeletal muscle gene expression in response to
      alternate day fasting," *Obesity Research* 13, no. 3 (2005): 574–81, https://
      pubmed.ncbi.nlm.nih.gov/15833943/.

154   *For women of reproductive age*: Rima Solianik et al., "Two-day fast-
      ing evokes stress, but does not affect mood, brain activity, cognitive,
      psychomotor, and motor performance in overweight women," *Be-
      havioural Brain Research* 338 (2018): 166–72, https://pubmed.ncbi
      .nlm.nih.gov/29097329/.

HACK 7: REACH FOR VINEGAR BEFORE YOU EAT

159   *By adding vinegar before meals for three months*: Tomoo Kondo et al.,
      "Vinegar intake reduces body weight, body fat mass, and serum tri-
      glyceride levels in obese Japanese subjects," *Bioscience, Biotechnology,
      and Biochemistry* 73, no. 8 (2009): 1837–43, https://www.tandfonline
      .com/doi/pdf/10.1271/bbb.90231.

159   *By adding vinegar before meals for three months*: Heitor O. Santos et al., "Vinegar (acetic acid) intake on glucose metabolism: A narrative review," *Clinical Nutrition ESPEN* 32 (2019): 1–7, https://www.research gate.net/publication/333526775_Vinegar_acetic_acid_intake_on_glu cose_metabolism_A_narrative_review.

159   *In one study, both groups were put on a strict weight-loss diet*: Solaleh Sadat Khezri et al., "Beneficial effects of Apple Cider Vinegar on weight management, Visceral Adiposity Index and lipid profile in overweight or obese subjects receiving restricted calorie diet: A randomized clinical trial," *Journal of Functional Foods* 43 (2018): 95–102, https:// www.sciencedirect.com/science/article/abs/pii/S1756464618300483.

159   *A Brazilian research team explained that*: Santos, "Vinegar (acetic acid) intake," 1–7.

159   *In nondiabetics, insulin-resistant people, people with type 1 or type 2 diabetes alike*: Farideh Shishehbor et al., "Vinegar consumption can attenuate postprandial glucose and insulin responses; a systematic review and meta-analysis of clinical trials," *Diabetes Research and Clinical Practice* 127 (2017): 1–9, https://www.researchgate.net /publication/314200733_Vinegar_consumption_can_attenuate_post prandial_glucose_and_insulin_responses_a_systematic_review_and _meta-analysis_of_clinical_trials.

159   *In nondiabetics, insulin-resistant people, people with type 1 or type 2 diabetes alike*: Santos, "Vinegar (acetic acid) intake," 1–7.

159   *The effects are also seen in women with PCOS*: Di Wu et al., "Intake of vinegar beverage is associated with restoration of ovulatory function in women with polycystic ovary syndrome," *The Tohoku Journal of Experimental Medicine* 230, no. 1 (2013): 17–23, https://www.jstage.jst .go.jp/article/tjem/230/1/230_17/_article/-char/ja/.

159   *The amount of insulin also decreases*: Panayota Mitrou et al., "Vinegar consumption increases insulin-stimulated glucose uptake by the forearm muscle in humans with type 2 diabetes," *Journal of Diabetes Research* (2015), https://www.hindawi.com/journals/jdr/2015/175204/.

161   *Scientists have found that the acetic acid*: Santos, "Vinegar (acetic acid) intake," 1–7.

161   *Second, once acetic acid gets into the bloodstream*: Santos, "Vinegar (acetic acid) intake," 1–7.

161   *It tells our DNA to reprogram*: Santos, "Vinegar (acetic acid) intake," 1–7.

161   *Reach for vinegar first*: Elin Östman et al., "Vinegar supplementation lowers glucose and insulin responses and increases satiety after a bread

meal in healthy subjects," *European Journal of Clinical Nutrition* 59, no. 9 (2005): 983–88, https://www.nature.com/articles/1602197/.

163   *In the first ever study looking at vinegar*: F. Brighenti et al., "Effect of neutralized and native vinegar on blood glucose and acetate responses to a mixed meal in healthy subjects," *European Journal of Clinical Nutrition* 49, no. 4 (1995): 242–47, https://pubmed.ncbi.nlm.nih .gov/7796781/.

163   *Vinegar to curb a glucose spike is most useful*: Stavros Liatis et al., "Vinegar reduces postprandial hyperglycaemia in patients with type II diabetes when added to a high, but not to a low, glycaemic index meal," *European Journal of Clinical Nutrition* 64, no. 7 (2010): 727–32, https:// www.nature.com/articles/ejcn201089.

167   *No studies have been done to measure the effects*: Santos, "Vinegar (acetic acid) intake," 1–7.

167   *Vinegar does not appear to damage the stomach lining*: Santos, "Vinegar (acetic acid) intake," 1–7.

167   *A 29-year-old woman who consumed 16 tablespoons of vinegar*: Santos, "Vinegar (acetic acid) intake," 1–7.

167   *Drinking it after eating*: Kondo, "Vinegar intake," 1837–43.

167   *When it comes to vinegar pills*: Carol S. Johnston et al., "Examination of the antiglycemic properties of vinegar in healthy adults," *Annals of Nutrition and Metabolism* 56, no. 1 (2010): 74–79, https://www.karger .com/Article/Abstract/272133.

167   *When it comes to vinegar pills*: Carol S. Johnston et al., "Preliminary evidence that regular vinegar ingestion favorably influences hemoglobin A1c values in individuals with type 2 diabetes mellitus," *Diabetes Research and Clinical Practice* 84, no. 2 (2009): e15–e17, https://www .sciencedirect.com/science/article/abs/pii/S0168822709000813.

HACK 8: AFTER YOU EAT, MOVE

171   *The more and the harder a muscle*: Erik A. Richter et al., "Exercise, GLUT4, and skeletal muscle glucose uptake," *Physiological Reviews* (2013), https://journals.physiology.org/doi/full/10.1152/physrev .00038.2012?view=long&pmid=23899560.

171   *It can increase 1,000-fold*: Julien S. Baker et al., "Interaction among skeletal muscle metabolic energy systems during intense exercise," *Journal of Nutrition and Metabolism* (2010), https://www.hindawi.com /journals/jnme/2010/905612/.

175 *Resistance exercise (weight lifting)*: Andrew Borror et al., "The effects of postprandial exercise on glucose control in individuals with type 2 diabetes: a systematic review," *Sports Medicine* 48, no. 6 (2018): 1479–91, https://link.springer.com/article/10.1007/s40279-018-0864-x.

175 *If our muscles are currently contracting*: Giovanni Messina et al., "Exercise causes muscle GLUT4 translocation in an insulin," *Biology and Medicine* 1 (2015): 1–4, https://www.researchgate.net/profile /Fiorenzo_Moscatelli/publication/281774994_Exercise_Causes_Muscle _GLUT4_Translocation_in_an_Insulin-Independent_Manner /links/55f7e0ee08aec948c474b805/Exercise-Causes-Muscle-GLUT4 -Translocation-in-an-Insulin-Independent-Manner.pdf.

175 *If our muscles are currently contracting*: Stephney Whillier, "Exercise and insulin resistance," *Advances in Experimental Medicine & Biology* 1228 (2020): 137–50, https://link.springer.com/chapter/10.1007 /978-981-15-1792-1_9.

176 *And the longer we work out*: Jason M. R. Gill., "Moderate exercise and post-prandial metabolism: issues of dose-response," *Journal of Sports Sciences* 20, no. 12 (2002): 961–67, https://shapeamerica.tandf online.com/doi/abs/10.1080/026404102321011715.

177 *Many different scenarios have been tested*: Sheri R. Colberg et al., "Postprandial walking is better for lowering the glycemic effect of dinner than pre-dinner exercise in type 2 diabetic individuals," *Journal of the American Medical Directors Association* 10, no. 6 (2009): 394–97, https://www.sciencedirect.com/science/article/abs/pii/S1525861 00900111X.

177 *In a study of resistance training*: Timothy D. Heden, "Postdinner resistance exercise improves postprandial risk factors more effectively than predinner resistance exercise in patients with type 2 diabetes," *Journal of Applied Physiology* 118, no. 5 (2015): 624–34, https://journals .physiology.org/doi/full/10.1152/japplphysiol.00917.2014.

177 *Among other things, it helps*: Heden, "Postdinner resistance exercise," 624–34.

177 *And reduces inflammation*: Sechang Oh et al., "Exercise reduces inflammation and oxidative stress in obesity-related liver diseases," *Medicine and Science in Sports and Exercise* 45, no. 12 (2013): 2214–22, https://pubmed.ncbi.nlm.nih.gov/23698242/.

177 *It'll be most impactful after meals*: Andrew N. Reynolds et al., "Advice to walk after meals is more effective for lowering postprandial

glycaemia in type 2 diabetes mellitus than advice that does not specify timing: a randomised crossover study," *Diabetologia* 59, no. 12 (2016): 2572–78, https://link.springer.com/article/10.1007/s00125-016-4085-2.

178 *The net effect of exercise is to reduce oxidative stress*: Sataro Goto et al., "Hormetic effects of regular exercise in aging: correlation with oxidative stress," *Applied Physiology, Nutrition, and Metabolism* 32, no. 5 (2007): 948–53, https://cdnsciencepub.com/doi/abs/10.1139/H07-092.

HACK 9: IF YOU HAVE TO SNACK, GO SAVORY

183 *That in people with this mental health condition*: Daphne Simeon et al., "Feeling unreal: a PET study of depersonalization disorder," *American Journal of Psychiatry* 157, no. 11 (2000): 1782–88, https://ajp.psychiatryonline.org/doi/full/10.1176/appi.ajp.157.11.1782.

183 *Science tells us that when people eat*: Kara L. Breymeyer et al., "Subjective mood and energy levels of healthy weight and overweight/obese healthy adults on high- and low-glycemic load experimental diets," *Appetite* 107 (2016): 253–59, https://pubmed.ncbi.nlm.nih.gov/27507131/.

183 *Science tells us that when people eat*: Rachel A. Cheatham et al., "Long-term effects of provided low and high glycemic load low energy diets on mood and cognition," *Physiology & Behavior* 98, no. 3 (2009): 374–79, https://pubmed.ncbi.nlm.nih.gov/19576915/.

183 *Science tells us that when people eat*: Sue Penckofer et al., "Does glycemic variability impact mood and quality of life?" *Diabetes Technology & Therapeutics* 14, no. 4 (2012): 303–10, https://www.ncbi.nlm.nih.gov/pmc/articles/PMC3317401/.

184 *The glucose in a candy or granola bar tends to go to storage*: Shimy, "Effects of dietary carbohydrate content on circulating metabolic fuel availability."

HACK 10: PUT SOME CLOTHES ON YOUR CARBS

187 *When you do enjoy carbs*: Nesti, "Impact of nutrient type," 144.

187 *Even savory snacks*: Lesley N. Lilly et al., "The effect of added peanut butter on the glycemic response to a high-glycemic index meal: A pilot study," *Journal of the American College of Nutrition* 38, no. 4 (2019): 351–57, https://pubmed.ncbi.nlm.nih.gov/30395790/.

187 *Even savory snacks*: David J. A. Jenkins et al., "Almonds decrease

postprandial glycemia, insulinemia, and oxidative damage in healthy individuals," *Journal of Nutrition* 136, no. 12 (2006): 2987–92, https://academic.oup.com/jn/article/136/12/2987/4663963.

188   *But the most recent science*: Nesti, "Impact of nutrient type," 144.

189   *Adding fat to a meal does not increase the insulin spike*: Gentilcore, "Effects of fat on gastric emptying," 2062–67.

189   *Eating carbohydrates alone isn't just*: Karen E. Foster-Schubert et al., "Acyl and total ghrelin are suppressed strongly by ingested proteins, weakly by lipids, and biphasically by carbohydrates," *Journal of Clinical Endocrinology & Metabolism* 93, no. 5 (2008): 1971–79, https://www.ncbi.nlm.nih.gov/pmc/articles/PMC2386677/.

190   *When we eat carbohydrates on their own*: Adapted from Foster-Schubert, "Acyl and total ghrelin," 1971–79.

191   *But thanks to a fascinating recent experiment*: Sabrina Strang et al., "Impact of nutrition on social decision making," *Proceedings of the National Academy of Sciences* 114, no. 25 (2017): 6510–14, https://www.pnas.org/content/114/25/6510/.

199   *Remember: when we combine glucose*: Nesti, "Impact of nutrient type," 144.

YOU ARE SPECIAL

219   *Starting in 2015, research teams*: Sarah E. Berry et al., "Human postprandial responses to food and potential for precision nutrition," *Nature Medicine* 26, no. 6 (2020): 964–73, https://www.nature.com/articles/s41591-020-0934-0.

220   *Some studies even found that if you* think: Chanmo Park et al., "Glucose metabolism responds to perceived sugar intake more than actual sugar intake," *Scientific Reports* 10, no. 1 (2020): 1–8, https://www.nature.com/articles/s41598-020-72501-w.

Index

continuous glucose monitors (CGMs) (*cont.*)
  graphs, *see* continuous glucose monitor (CGM) graphs
  inability to measure fructose and insulin, 7, 36–37
  operation of, 32
cookies, 179, 207, 220
Cornell University, 73, 81
coronavirus complications, 57
cravings, xxvii–xxviii, 5, 53, 55–56, 108
  artificial sweeteners and, 145–46
  breakfast and, 122
  cheat sheet, 205–7
  cooling-off period for, 205–6
  dopamine release and, 27, 29–30, 56, 143
  green starter and, 90–91, 96
  reducing, 148, 157
C-reactive protein, 64–65
C-section, 58
Crohn's disease, 63

dementia, 46, 61–62
depersonalization-derealization disorder, xxiii–xxiv, 181–83, 192
depression, 5, 62, 183, 191
dessert:
  food order for meals and, 85
  processed fruit as, 123–24
  sweet snacks vs., 149–55
  vinegar before or after eating, *see* vinegar / apple cider vinegar
diabetes:
  Alzheimer's as "type 3 diabetes," 61
  coma and, 109
  exercise after meals and, 175
  fasting glucose level and, 32–33
  food order for meals and, 73

gestational, 5, 57–58, 140–42
glucose spike levels for, 117
glycemic index and, 142
hemoglobin A1c (HbA1c) test, 46, 73, 193, 202
inflammation and, 46
prediabetes, 5, 32, 33, 62, 67, 117
reactive hypoglycemia and, 109
23andMe continuous glucose monitor study, xxv–xxvi
type 1, 5, 48, 59–60, 191–94, 202
type 2, *see* type 2 diabetes
diets and dieting:
  Atkins, 22
  gluten-free, 122, 215
  keto, 6, 22
  low-calorie, 68
  low fat, 68
  sustainable lifestyle vs., 6
  vegan, 6, 122, 215
  vegetarian, 110–11, 122
  see also calorie counting
diet soda, 144–45, 147
dinner, in sample menus, 112, 218
dizziness, 5, 53
DNA, 43, 62, 101, 161
dopamine release / pleasure, 27, 29–30, 56, 143
doughnuts, 103–4, 106, 182–83
dried fruit, 132, 138–41, 197
Duke University, 66

eczema, 60
eggs, 126, 128, 129, 130, 131, 136, 186, 193, 194, 196, 206, 207
energy crashes, 5
enzymes:
  alpha-amylase, 13–14, 18, 75–76, 161
  role of, 12, 13–16
erectile dysfunction, 66

About the Author

Jessie is on a mission to translate cutting-edge science into easy tips to help people improve their physical and mental health. She's the founder of the widely popular Instagram account @GlucoseGoddess, where she teaches hundreds of thousands about healthy food habits. She holds a bachelor of science degree in mathematics from King's College, London, and a master of science degree in biochemistry from Georgetown University. Her work at a genetic analysis start-up in Silicon Valley made her realize that, as the key to good health, food habits beat genetics. In this book, Jessie shares her startling discovery about the essential role of blood sugar in every aspect of our lives, from cravings to fertility, and the surprising hacks to optimize it while still eating the foods we love.